Mixed Nuts

Mixed Nuts

A novel

Suzanne D. Lonn

Suzanne D. Lonn

Author of the novel *The Game of Hearts*

To order additional copies of this book, contact:
Xlibris Corporation
1-888-795-4274
www.Xlibris.com
Orders@Xlibris.com
53904

CONTENTS

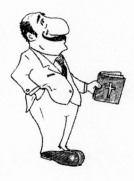

God has blessed me with close friendships with elderly people, and Mixed Nuts is dedicated to you, my older friends. I adore, revere, appreciate, and respect you. It is an honor to have you in my life. In fact, I need you in my life.

So, when I write about "mixed nuts," please don't be offended! I say it all "tongue-in-cheek" and with love, and after all, as my mother used to tell me, "We are all a little crazy, except for thee and me, and sometimes I wonder about thee!"

God bless all my friends!

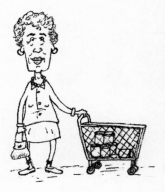

PROLOGUE

On a cold, October morning in 2007, when the icing of hoarfrost was still on the golf course, and the geese gathered on the greens and waited in the steamy meltdown of the night before, two old duffers ambled along the creek bank, looking for wayward golf balls. The white orbs, like small, frozen snowballs, lay hidden in the tall, marshy grass. It was a Sunday morning ritual for Jerry and Dave to search for errant balls. They took their time, whacking at the brush and overgrown weeds and occasionally bending over to pluck their prize.

It was too early in the day to play a round of golf, even though in southern Oregon, the remnants of summer often hang on into late autumn. By noon, the warm sun would melt the crystals on the course and tenderly kiss the foreheads of the diehard golfers, reminding them that it will come again next year, as blazing hot as ever.

But on that autumn morning, their scavenger hunt produced more than dimpled golf balls, and their eighteen holes on the course hung suspended in mid-air. A set of distinct footprints, like those of tennis shoes, was imprinted on the sloping creek bank. Nearby rested a small, amber-colored bottle—a medicine bottle. It was empty.

At the same time, Otis Lemming discovered the dead body of his twin brother, Oscar, in his bed at Pear Blossom Plaza Retirement Home, just a few yards from the creek and the golf course. Ordinarily, that would not be an unusual event, but the police were called when the back door, facing the creek, was discovered propped wide open, and the coroner requested an autopsy. Something was just not quite right.

"Well, I wasn't going to say anything, because I'm just an old woman, and nobody believes a nutty, old woman," Essie, said when she heard the news, "but late last night I saw a person in a black, leather jacket, standing by the creek. Oh, yes, it was leather all right; I could tell by the smoothness and the way the light of the full moon hit it, and then I saw a shovel and . . ."

CHAPTER ONE

Seasoned with Salt

"We's all poor nuts
And things happen
And we yust get
Mixed in wrong,
That's all."
—Eugene O'Neill

They come and they go. The residential registry changes like the seasons. Some leave, for one reason or another, before they unpack all their boxes; others go away unexpectedly and forever, where no baggage is required.

They come from all over the state of Oregon, across county lines, from down the street or across the town of Middleford. Some have come up I-5 from California or over from the Pacific Coast, all to live together at Pear Blossom Plaza.

The sixty residents are similar in so many ways and yet so uniquely different in their personalities and problems. One day they can't stand each other, and the next, they are sitting together around the game table "workin' the puzzle" or tapping their toes and smiling at Josie, who is playing hymns on the organ.

They reside and they mingle together like the ordinary peanut and the distinguished cashew in a can of mixed nuts. The walnuts and almonds and filberts add flavor and flair to the mix.

Lightly salted, honey-coated, dry roasted, mixed and shaken together . . . Mixed Nuts!

*   *   *

A new resident had never arrived at Pear Blossom Retirement Home in a flashy, red convertible, so naturally, the two senior sentinels stationed voluntarily just inside the front door were clueless as to who was actually pulling up into the drop-off spot in front of the building. The U-Haul appeared first, and the driver drove a little beyond the entrance, followed by the sports car.

"It must be the grandkid's car. I hear she has nine of them," Bertha wisely informed Antonio, as she perched on the edge of her wheelchair.

Antonio nodded diplomatically in agreement. He'd learned early on in his tenure not to argue with Bertha; she knew it all, and if she didn't, she'd be right there in the office in the morning to try to find out. He stood up from the seat of his *Cadillac,* as he called his fancy walker to get a better vantage point. "I hear she's seventy-eight," he added.

"Oh, she is not! Where did you hear that? She's seventy-nine, and if you don't believe me, just ask her. There now! Look! That must be Maria getting out of the car."

A short, plump, elderly lady slowly pulled her body up from the enveloping bucket seat, grabbing onto any available handle for assistance.

"Three, two, one! We have lift-off," her daughter, Caterina quipped. She hurried around from the driver's side to help launch her mother.

"I just hate these low-slung cars! They're not for old people, and when you put the top down, my hair just goes to pot," the old lady grumbled, as her red shoes hit the pavement. "I'm just too old and too crippled up to try to get in and out. I wish you had a van or a sedan with a hard top."

Caterina grimaced. "Sorry, Mom, but I love my car."

Maria turned and reached into the bucket-seat to grab her purse that matched her shoes, and then, turning back toward her daughter, stood for a moment to get her bearings. "It was fun, though, when we'd take drives over to the coast, and you'd put the top down. Nobody knew me there, so I didn't care if I looked wind-blown." She smiled and looked up at her daughter. "Can we do it again some day?" she asked wistfully, fluffing her dyed, permed hair with her fingers.

"Yes, Mom, our good times are not over yet. It's still February, but come June, we'll run over and see the ocean. Try to be patient." Caterina knew that was like trying to calm the waves or tell the wind to stop blowing, but it had to be said.

Maria's smile disappeared as quickly as it had come, and the seventy-eight-year-old lady drew in a deep breath. "You know, this is like being in labor. You wish you'd never gotten to that point of no return, and it's so painful, but it's too late to back out, so you just bear it. So, come on. Let's give birth to this new life of mine, and go on in, and see the apartment." She grabbed Caterina's arm, more so for moral support than walking assistance. She straightened herself up to try to look taller than her five feet, thrust out her chin with all the determination she could muster, and squinted at the door that was magically swinging open. The robber of eyesight, macular degeneration, was one of the reasons she couldn't live alone any longer, so she really couldn't see Antonio or Bertha or know that they had pushed the automatic door-opener.

The clanging of the U-Haul door being raised in the background nearly drowned out Antonio's greeting. "Welcome to Pear Blossom. You must be Maria. I'm Antonio and this is Bertha," gushed the kindly, white-haired, old gentleman, as he offered his hand.

Maria didn't like to shake germy hands, so she kept one hand through her daughter's arm and the other one in the pocket of her white rain jacket. "Nice to meet you both," Maria said cordially. Then she noticed his walker with a dirty washcloth hanging over the basket, and she saw Bertha's wheelchair.

Have I come to this? she thought, as she gripped Caterina's arm even tighter. As they skirted the wheeled conveyances and headed through the lobby, they heard Bertha call out, "Your apartment is the first one next to the library."

Then she heard Antonio's deep booming voice "And Maria, Friday night is the potluck and I'm bringing my famous chili. Be sure to come. You'll see the sign-up sheet on the bulletin board, but since you're new here, you don't have to bring anything this time."

Maria's hand shot to her mouth as if she was going to be sick. "I'd never touch a thing that man cooked. To be frank with you, they'll never see me at a potluck! What's his name?" she whispered, as she fumbled for her apartment key.

"I think it is Chili Bob," Caterina had forgotten it, too.

*   *   *

Maria's son, Michael and his twin boys, Brian and Darren, quickly moved the boxes into her apartment. The hours that Cat and Maria envisioned unpacking slowly and methodically melted away quickly with Jillian, Michael's wife, assigning jobs, and most of Maria's possessions were nestled in their proper little niches before the sun had time to set.

"Here, boys, put these dishes in the kitchen cupboards. Michael, fill the pantry with the canned goods, the ironing board, and the clothes hamper. Cat, you can work in the bathroom, and Maria, where do you want the hide-a-bed that will be delivered any minute?"

The queen-sized hide-a-bed was delivered promptly on schedule at 4:00 in the afternoon. The family all agreed it was far too big for the size of the apartment, but Maria insisted that she had to keep it for overnight guests. "Cat, get the sheets on it; you're the one sleeping here tonight, and you can test the firmness. It's a six-inch mattress, you know."

Cat was so exhausted she could have slept on a pallet, and when the others left for their home on the hill, Cat and Maria barely had enough energy to brush their teeth. So, when there was a knock on the door that evening, they ignored it. "It's probably someone who has lost her way home," Maria grumbled, as she washed her bottom teeth and put them away for the night. "Don't they know they could have scared me, and I could have dropped my teeth in the sink?"

The next morning they found hanging from the door handle a tiny, heart-shaped basket full of Hershey kisses. The tiny gift card said, "Welcome, from the bottom of my heart."

"Oh, Mom has a sweetie already," Cat teased her mother. "It must be from Chili Bob; he's the only man you've met so far, and Valentine's Day is just around the corner. He's starting early."

"Whoever it is can just stop! I have enough to deal with without being bothered by a man! The only man I want to see right now is the maintenance man, so I can get these curtains hung!" Her voice rose higher and louder as her request became known, and with that cue, Cat scurried off to find the man with the ladder and his tools.

A man in a blue jump-suit with keys dangling from his belt and a hammer in his hand was hanging a large picture in the lobby.

"Hi there," Cat said cheerily. "Are you the maintenance man?" Cat asked, as she put out her hand to shake his. "I'm Cat, and my mother just moved into Apartment 101."

"Sure am. The name is Tony. Sorry, my hands are full, but how can I help you?"

"Well, my mother has some draperies she would like you to hang," Cat stated her mother's request.

Tony answered as he secured the picture in place on the wall. "I'm sorry, but you'll have to tell your mother that she has to live with the drapes that are already there." He shrugged his shoulders. "There's nothing I can do about it."

Cat nodded, not surprised at his answer. "Could you tell her? She wants to talk to you about some light bulbs, too."

"Sure. I'm used to this. Besides working here, I have family here." He winked at Cat, squared his broad shoulders, and marched off to Maria's apartment, ready to take the blame.

Cat, meanwhile, took that time for herself, and looked around the facility. The four washing machines were humming a tune in the laundry room just off the lobby in the west wing of the main floor, and one lady was watching Reverend Robert Schuller in the library/tv room, adjacent to Maria's apartment on the east side. All was dark and quiet in the Community Room, as Cat made her way past the tables that often teemed with hot dishes and salads, and Chili Bob's recipe. The puzzle on the game table was waiting patiently for someone to add another piece, and the organ in the corner by the door was silent, awaiting young Josie's arrival for the Wednesday evening sing-a-long.

Cat was enjoying the fresh air on the patio when she noticed cigarette butts and a half-smoked and still-lit cigar smoldering in an ash tray on a patio table. She looked around and saw nobody to claim it, so she buried it in the dirt in an empty hanging planter.

"Put it out; it's making an ash of itself." Maria had arrived on the scene.

"So, how did it go with the M and M?" Cat inquired.

"The what? Who?" Maria was puzzled.

"The maintenance man."

"Well, I have to live with the drapes that are there, and just like I surmised, he doesn't normally work on Sundays, so I have to fill out a request, turn it in, and he has to come back, and fix my ceiling lights. You'd think when a new person moves in, everything would be in tip-top shape, wouldn't you? And why was he even in the building if he doesn't work on Sundays? So many mysteries and such folderol!!"

Cat tried to clear up the mystery. "He has family here. That's what he told me."

As they wandered on around the corner of the building, they could see the creek bed just below and on the opposite side of that, the golf course.

"What a view you have, Mom!"

The living room and bedroom windows of Maria's apartment afforded a picture-perfect setting.

"I really wanted to be on the other side, so I could see the parking lot and people coming and going, but I guess it doesn't matter; I can't see too well anyway," Maria said sadly.

"This side of the building will be a lot cooler in the summer. You'll have the morning sun, but not the heat in the afternoon, and look, there are the garden boxes. I wonder how you go about getting your name on one of those. Mom, you could have flowers and a tomato plant," Cat added cheerily.

"Another thing to check on when the office opens up in the morning. I'll have to start a list. Maybe you can do that when we get back to my room, dear."

"I will, but Mom, let's try to remember not to call it your *room*. It's your *apartment*."

"Oh well, whatever. Let's go back to my palatial mansion. I forgot to take my pills, and I never forget those. This moving just has me all off schedule."

As Maria and Cat neared the patio table and chairs, they saw two men sitting and smoking. Cat recognized them right away, but Maria couldn't make out their faces until she was practically upon them. Squinting only blocked out the sun.

The older gentleman politely stood and offered his hand to Maria, as he had done the day before. "Good morning, ladies," Antonio said.

"Oh hello, Chili . . . Chilly out this morning, isn't it?" Maria recovered, plunging her hands deeply into her coat pocket. "Germs *and* nicotine! A lethal combination!" she muttered under her breath.

"There is a refreshing nip in the air," noted Antonio, dismissing what she had said. "Oh, I almost forgot. I would like you to meet my son, Tony. He is the maintenance man here. You might need to call on him some day."

"We've already met," the trio said in perfect harmony, and Tony winked at Cat for the second time that morning.

"I wonder if M and M is married," Cat whispered to her mother, as they entered the door and went through the Community Room.

"Are you always going to call him that?" Maria chided. "He has a name now. Besides, you don't want to get mixed up with him. It's too soon after your divorce . . . What's that noise?"

"Sounds like the spin cycle to me. There are four washing machines going all at once."

"What? These old people are washing clothes on the Lord's Day? Why aren't they in church?"

Suddenly realizing she wasn't filling a pew either, she added, "Oh, well, cleanliness *is* next to godliness."

* * *

After a relaxing Sunday afternoon of just puttering around the apartment and rearranging dishes and cookware in the kitchen and towels and cosmetics in the bathroom to suit Maria's whims, mother and daughter planned their week.

"I really should think about going home one of these days," Cat remarked. "After all, I have been away for two weeks helping you pack and clean and get moved down here."

"What? You're just going to dump me and run? I thought you'd stay at least a few days and help me get acquainted with these new neighbors of mine, and we could ride around the city and see what all has changed since I was here visiting. Mostly I need to find a good pharmacy and a good mocha stand. Please stay awhile. Oh, please stay, Cat."

Cat could hear tears in her mother's voice, and she knew she should stay on a little longer.

"I didn't mean right away, Mom. It was just a thought for the future," Cat tried to assuage her mother's fears. "I know you must be overwhelmed by the move and all the new people in your life. You know . . . I could use a mocha right now. Let's go see if there's a coffee stand close by."

Cat soon pulled up to the drive-in window of Beans on Barnett, and Maria gave Cat the instructions for her drink. "I want a 16 ounce, iced mocha, single shot, with whipped cream, and no bean. It sticks to my mouth, you know."

"Yes, I know," Cat sighed and threw out a challenge. "Someday you should try a Mt. Shasta Almond Joy or a Rogue River Rumble. Take a bold step where no Mom has gone before."

"Oh, you're so funny, but in all your hilarity, you forgot to order napkins," Maria chided.

They did have fun together. Maria laughed, as Cat, with her tongue, chased a coffee bean that was drowning in the whipped cream of her Granita. Cat listened with rapt attention to her mother as she mentally searched her recipe files for a dish to take to the potluck that she "was never going to attend."

"If you'll stay for the potluck, I'll go, but just this once, . . . please. After all, it is a Valentine's Day potluck, and don't you want to be with your mother on Valentine's Day?"

Such bribery, Cat thought to herself, but she did realize that she should stay a few more days and help Mom through this painful and uncertain transition from being totally on her own to adapting to a new life with strangers and unfamiliar surroundings.

"I had a feeling you'd go to the potluck. Chili Bob, I mean Antonio, would be so disappointed if you didn't show up," Cat teased. "You won't need me, but yes, I'll stay and we'll go." This would give Mom an incentive to live happily for a few more days.

"I can live without Antonio," Maria snorted, "but I don't know if I can live without you. The ones I've met so far look like a bunch of mixed nuts to me!"

PEAR BLOSSOM PLAZA
OFFICIAL BULLETIN BOARD

Sign-up Sheet
For Potluck
February 14, 2007

	NAME:	FOOD ITEM:
1.	Millie	Cheese curls
2.	Sarah	Baked chicken
3.	Bertha	Garden Salad
4.	Essie	Green Salad
5.	Antonio	Chili
6.	Winnie	Red jello or green
7.	Otis	Olives and Pickles
8.	Oscar	Pickled beets and little corn cobs
9.	B.K.	(Don't know yet)
10.	Maria	Cannoli
11.	Gayle	Green Bean Casserole

NEED MORE HOT DISHES!!

Lost!!
My scissors.
The ones I use to cut up my chickens.

Last seen in my Bible.

Return to Essie, RM. 120

Bus trip to Wal Mart
Monday, Feb. 17. 10:00 A.M.

DON'T FORGET!
Sing-along-with Josie on
Wednesday night 7:00 p.m.

Association Meeting Thurs.
Night at 6:30

KOFFEE KLATCH

Saturday 9:30 a.m.

To be rescheduled.
Notice from Office:
Please put all lost and found notices
on resident's bulletin board around
the corner—not this one!!

Bible Study Wed. 1:30 in library.
All are welcome.
Sit and swivel exercise class on Wed.
canceled, due to Bible study at the
same time to be rescheduled.

CHAPTER TWO

Sarah's Soliloquy

"As a white candle
In a holy place,
So is the beauty
Of an aged face."
—Joseph Campbell

"Oh, dear! Imagine me at ninety-three and still having hot flashes! What to do . . . oh, what to do? Well, during the day when I'm here all alone, I'll just unbutton my blouse and throw it back over my shoulders. Of course, I'll leave it tucked in at the back in case someone taps on my door, and I have to answer it in a hurry."

Sarah stared at the aging lady in the mirror of her dressing table. She pushed back from her forehead the white tendrils of her short perm and bent her sore back closer for better inspection. The mirror, which was easily as old as she was, stared back in silence.

"Oh, well. So what if the doctor says I'll flash 'til I'm under the sod; I still have my beautiful, shapely legs—my gams. Everyone says so," she announced, as she rubbed one calf and then the other. "And the doctor says I still have all my marbles, too!"

She was tired and looked drawn and pale. It had been another restless night. The hot flashes were at their hottest then—a swift and intense heating of the entire body, followed in due time by a slow, cooling trend. It sounded like a weather report or maybe this was what was meant by global warming!

She'd talked to Bertha who lived downstairs about it. Bertha was reputed to know everything, but Sarah had gotten no satisfaction from her. Bertha told her to turn the heat down and open a window. "You know they keep this place too hot in the winter and too cold in the summer," Bertha advised. She'd acted like it was physically impossible for a ninety-three year-old woman to have hot flashes and even alluded to the fact that it was all in Sarah's head. From then on, Sarah decided that Bertha didn't know everything. She had even said that global warming was a scam. Imagine that!

"Well, I'll just commiserate with the new lady in 101. She might have good, common sense. Lord only knows; We need someone with some sense around here!" Sarah went on talking to the mirror. "Now, what was her name?"

Sarah often proclaimed loudly and clearly and with great dramatic flair that she did not like to talk. "Well, you know I don't," she'd try to convince her daughter and her best friends, but, since they couldn't get a word in to contradict her, they just politely agreed, smirking all the while. That irritated her just as much as if they'd argued with her, and she would repeat herself, "Now come on; you know I don't like to talk. If I see someone getting out of the elevator, I just turn and go the other way. I don't want to talk to them. You see, they're all old people around here."

*   *   *

Sarah had the important duty each evening at 7:00 to pick up the daily newspaper from the library. She was as devoted to this job as a dog is to his master, and she even gave up watching *Jeopardy* to fulfill her obligation on time. After all, the members of The Association had voted and assigned her this task, and she felt it was an honor bestowed upon her and not to be taken lightly. She kept the newspapers in her apartment until she had two or three day's worth and then carried them outside and down the sidewalk to the recycling bin.

"Oh, my goodness, it's time, and it's the big paper today." Sarah remarked to herself on that particular Sunday evening. "I wonder who I'll see out in the lobby tonight. Maybe the new lady?" And off she trotted to gather up the *Middleford Valley View*.

Sarah had lived in Middleford her entire life. She was now a widow with one grown daughter living in Iowa, and she had a myriad of friends. A bridge player for years, a professional book reviewer, and a librarian at the local library had given her access to the public arena, and she knew a variety of people in all walks of life. In spite of her adamant assertion of "not liking to talk," she was well-known around the community for her public speaking abilities, her sense of humor, and her downright good old-fashioned friendliness. She was called upon to give book reviews whenever The Friends of the Library needed some entertainment at their business meetings or at the Civic Club Tea or a church social. Why, just last week a lady had called from the Ann Miller Theater asking Sarah to review the book, *The Da Vinci Code*. Regrettably, Sarah had turned them down, stating that she and that book "did not get along too well together." She suggested some of her favorites, but, no, the members of the Middleford Study Club were insistent on that book. Sarah advised them to call another time.

*   *   *

The lobby was humming with activity as Sarah rounded up the portions of the Sunday paper from the library. Several ladies were chatting in the overstuffed chairs around the periphery of the lobby, and Bertha was holding court in the center near the huge, flower arrangement. The ladies under her spell were listening with rapt attention as Bertha shared her concerns of misconduct of the residents that had taken place over the weekend. They were nodding in agreement, and they knew that first thing Monday morning, Bertha would assert her authority and "take care of business" in the administrator's office, as she did every Monday without fail and sometimes later in the week if infractions continued.

The most vile offense that had happened since Bertha became the self-appointed judge and jury had taken place again last night. Essie, Bertha's most prized spy, had reported that once again late at night, Betty had gone out in front with her pomeranian and allowed the dog to relieve herself down the drainage grate in the driveway near the entrance.

Bertha sat up straight in her wheelchair to full authority. "I'll take care of it first thing in the morning; don't you worry. Either that woman or her dog or both will have to go!"

Nodding in agreement, the women shuffled off to check out the bulletin boards before retiring for the night. The messages were posted on the wall across from the library, and Sarah was pleased that she had taken her time gathering the papers and even straightening a few book shelves. I love old people, she thought as she listened to their chatter about the menu for the potluck. She hoped the gaggle of geese would approve of her contribution.

"Millie is bringing cheese curls again. What a lazy tightwad! How hard is it to dump some snacks into a bowl?"

"As usual, B.K. doesn't write out her name, like it is some secret code and we don't know it's Betty, and look, she doesn't even know what to bring. How can we plan what we are bringing when she doesn't even tell us what she is doing? She gets on my last nerve!"

Sarah sat at a table in the library pretending to read a magazine and listened to their complaints.

They soon came to her name. "Well, at least Sarah has some good sense and is bringing baked chicken. Lord knows, we never get enough meat, just Antonio's chili, and it's too spicy for me!"

Sarah was pleased with herself and their approval, when suddenly, she heard a voice she didn't recognize. She scooted around in her chair and craned her neck to see better.

Oh, I bet it's the new lady. She spotted two unfamiliar faces, one younger than the other, who was reading the menu to the older lady. Oh yes, I heard her daughter was here for a few days, Sarah nodded to herself, and I heard she's a writer, too.

"Why is Antonio bringing chili? I thought he was Italian." Maria asked of no one in particular but everyone in general.

They all laughed and told Maria and Cat that he always, without fail, brings chili. "You must be new around here or you'd know that . . . oh, are you *The New Lady*?" Winnie asked.

"Chili Bob, remember?" Cat whispered to her mother, who gave Cat a knowing smile in return.

"Yes, I'm *The New Lady*, and my name is Maria and this is my daughter Cat."

"Oh, that's an odd name. Does she live her, too?" Winnie seemed to have become the spokesman for the group. Her face was so wrinkled she looked like she'd slept in it.

"No, she helped me move in and she'll be here for a few more days." The women seemed more interested in Cat than in Maria. They eyed her up and down and patted her on the back. Cat's dimples and friendly smile were their reward.

Winnie continued her interrogation for the group. "Are you both coming to the potluck? You need to sign up if you are."

Maria sighed at Winnie's ignorance and lack of attention to detail. "Well, I guess so; See, I already signed up!"

With the tip of her cane, Winnie went down the list on the bulletin board. "Cannoli? What in the world is that? We don't do fancy dishes around here."

Maria could see that; Winnie was bringing Jello, red or green.

"I know what it is!" Sarah could contain herself no longer and popped out of the library, scattering her pile of newspapers on the floor as she bustled up to Maria. "Don't you ladies ever watch *Everybody Loves Raymond?*" Marie is always making cannoli for her boys, and this is Maria, like Marie. Don't you ladies get the connection? I bet you like that show, don't you, Maria? Oh, I haven't met you yet. My name is Sarah. I heard you were coming and had moved into 101 and I've been so anxious to meet you. Of course, I know how it is when you move. There's so much to do and put away and arrange and rearrange and it can take days. Oh, where are my manners? You must be the daughter. My daughter lives in Iowa and that's so far away. Where are you from?" Sarah finally came up for breath and extended her hand first to Maria and then to Cat.

The other ladies knew their time had run out and Sarah had taken over. "But, what is cannoli?" they wondered, as they wandered down the hall.

"Look it up in the dictionary; it will give you something to do!" Sarah called to them.

Winnie turned and shook her antique cane at Sarah.

"Look out for her, you two," Sarah continued. "She has a flask in the top of that cane and she often sneaks a shot. Then she gets mean. Now that is something Bertha could report! But she won't because they are both busybodies. Well, who am I to talk? I don't even like to talk! By the way, what is cannoli? I mean, what is it really? I've never really known. Marie serves it on that sitcom, but she never says what's in it. You know, I don't really like sitcoms; all that laughter in the background, canned or live, really bothers me!"

Maria grabbed Cat's arm for support as Sarah rattled on. "Why don't you come down in the morning for coffee and I'll show you the cannoli recipe and see what you think. Maybe it is too fancy for the folks around here. It's just one of many foods that we Italians like, and I wanted to bring something special for my first potluck." Maria surprised even herself with her excitement.

"I accept with alacrity, as long as I don't have to come too early. Oft times I don't sleep well in the night, but then around dawn, I sleep better. I'm in a bad way."

Maria suggested 10:00 a.m. as a reasonable hour, and that pleased Sarah. "10:00 it is! I'm anxious to see your apartment; I bet it is fixed up cute!" Sarah bubbled with as much anticipation as if she had been invited to have high tea with the Queen of England.

"Cat and I are still rearranging. You wouldn't think that for such a small place it would be so hard to decide where to put things," Maria offered.

Sarah agreed. "Before I moved in, I had a garage sale, so that helped weed out what I knew I wouldn't want, but I still brought utensils I'll never use, such as a meat grinder. Now when do you think I will ever use a meat grinder?"

They all laughed and agreed some things just take up space. Cat was inching her way down the hall and trying to get away, and Maria was making her move that direction, too.

"We've got to go, but we'll see you in the morning," Maria said, stifling a yawn.

"9:30 it is." Sarah waved good night.

Cat and Maria frowned at each other simultaneously. "I thought we agreed on 10:00. Oh well, whenever she gets there is okay. We need to get some things done in the afternoon, Cat. I must find a good pharmacist, and I must get the ingredients for whatever I am making for the potluck. It'll be a busy day tomorrow, I can tell that right now, so put out the Cat and lock the door." They loved to say that to each other and had for many years. Maria got tears in her eyes when she thought that soon Cat would be gone, and she'd be alone.

Cat, who never missed much, noticed the misty eyes. "What's up, Mom?"

"I don't want to say that any more. I don't want to put you out, and I don't want to be alone when you leave."

"Well, what has happened to my tough, brave, independent little mom? You've always been able to tackle the world and all it's problems. And you won't be alone. You're surrounded by . . ."

"Yeah, surrounded by mixed nuts! Say, maybe we should get a can of mixed nuts and take them to the potluck." Maria tried hard to get the sparkle back in her eyes and end the day with a joke.

"Funny, Mom, but no one would get the humor, and it would just be one step up from Millie and her cheese curls."

"Oh, did we meet Millie?" Maria puzzled. "Hmm . . . No, I think she is the one, though, that was an actress at one time. I heard someone talking about her and how she insists that we should get a Jacuzzi. Can you imagine in a place like this? This is HUD housing, not The Trump Towers!"

"If she was an actress, why is she living in a place like this?" Cat's inquisitive mind was quick to wonder.

"Maybe she was just a wannabe. All I know is that right now, all I wannabe is to be in bed."

"Me, too, Mom. Catch you on the other side of midnight."

A good night kiss and hug and Maria fell into bed, while Cat bedded down in the living room. They were both too tired to hear the ruckus in the lobby.

CHAPTER THREE

The Twins

"I wish I loved the human race;
I wish I loved its silly face;
I wish I liked the way it walks;
I wish I liked the way it talks;
And when I'm introduced to one,
I wish I thought, 'What jolly fun!'"
—Wishes of an elderly man.
Sir Walter Raleigh

Thin, dark blue sweaters stretched over hunched backs decorated with flakes of dandruff, brown but graying hair combed neatly and identically, blue slacks with bulging pleats at the waistlines, and black lace-up shoes with big, rounded toes was the continual daily attire of the twins, Oscar and Otis Lemming. Boring and predictable, shy and quiet, and lonely and unto themselves characterized their dispositions. The two retired mailmen had lived at Pear Blossom Plaza for a year and virtually knew no one. The only functions they attended were the potlucks and the Association Meetings, and at each event they sat quietly, never mingling or offering a clue as to what was running through their minds.

The rumor mill spit out the idea that Oscar was sweet on Millie and was secretly courting her, but she denied it vehemently. "How disgusting!" She nearly gagged each time someone teased her about it, but one Monday morning she couldn't deny that she had been with Oscar the night before when he fell as they came in the front door together. She insisted that it didn't prove anything; they just happened to be coming in at the same time, but then she made the mistake of embellishing her story by describing the chocolate sundaes at Dairy

Queen. How did she get there? She didn't drive, but Otis and Oscar still had a car. The gossips surely picked up the ball and ran with that one!

Millie had fussed over Oscar until the medics arrived and had given him the once-over and pronounced him fit and unharmed in any way. As he shuffled off to the apartment he shared with Otis, the wags in the lobby whispered, "Did you see how he fell for her?"

The gossip continued and picked up speed Monday morning, and as Bertha waited in her wheelchair for the office to open up, she heard several versions and exaggerations.

For once she had missed something going on in the lobby and she felt terrible about that. "Slept right through it, I guess. Why didn't someone alert me?" She snorted in disgust, to all who tried to clue her in to the alleged antics of Millie and Oscar. Now she'd have to sort it all out, sift the chaff from the wheat, and come to a conclusion. She didn't have time for any more crises; Monday mornings were her busiest times of the entire week.

With documentation in hand of the weekend's grievances, she waited even more impatiently than usual for Sherrie, the administrator, to turn on the lights and unlock the door.

"I think she is hiding back there behind her desk, not wanting to talk to me, and I can't imagine why she wouldn't want to hear me out when I am the only one who really knows what goes on around here on the weekends, and I give her the straight scoop, too!" Bertha continued her monologue to Antonio, who was waiting for the Metro van.

Nodding in agreement, Antonio said, "Yes, I saw her come in the back door when I went out for a smoke and that was thirty minutes ago, but she is so nice; I can't imagine her making you wait unless she got tied up on the phone or stuck on the computer."

Bertha was even more impatient. "To think she wouldn't open the door first is a crying shame!"

Just then, they heard the click of the lock and the office door swung open. Sherrie's face lit up like a billboard, and the warmth she exuded could melt even Bertha's cold heart. That was Sherrie's motive on Monday mornings: "Kill them with kindness," her mother had taught her, and it set the tone for her dealings with the residents for the entire week.

Sherrie's demeanor really was genuine, and although she dreaded Monday mornings and Bertha's laundry list of the weekend's infractions, she handled herself and the residents and their problems with grace and dignity. Most felt her love and caring heart, and they knew she was there to help them through their uncertain time at Pear Blossom Plaza.

"Good morning, Bertha. Come on in and have a cup of coffee and let's chat. How was the weekend?" Sherrie hoped against hope that it was quiet.

"I'm not here for coffee; I have a busy morning. Something unexpected has come up, and I have to investigate it." Bertha cut right to the chase. "I don't suppose you heard about what happened last night with Oscar and Millie."

"Yes, I was briefed on it this morning by my assistant, but all turned out well, so let's begin with your list." Sherrie was anxious to bypass that subject and move on.

"I trust that you are really going to do something about the dog situation this time. You say that you will talk to the owners', but I just wonder if you really do. Betty still allows that rat of a dog to pee down the drainage ditch. It happened again over the weekend, and at night when you aren't here to see it." Bertha's dander was up, and she was red in the face.

"And that's not all; Gayle's dog upchucked right in front of the elevator on the carpet."

"Did Gayle clean it up?" Sherrie asked.

"Oh, she swiped at it and spritzed something on it." Bertha downplayed any attempts of others capabilities and attempts to right their wrongs.

"As you know, Bertha, the poor dog couldn't help it. You know how terrified she is of the elevator. Gayle usually carries her in her arms when she comes through the lobby and gets on the elevator, and that calms the dog and nothing happens."

"Well, her arms were full of groceries, but that's no excuse. She should have carried the dog up first. That's what I would have done." Bertha stated indignantly.

"I'll check out the carpet and see if it's stained, and then remind her to carry the dog through the lobby and onto the elevator. It was just an accident and those do happen. As for the other dog problem, I'll tell Betty to take the dog out the back door and have it use the designated area. That should take care of it."

"I doubt it," Bertha grumbled. "If it doesn't, I will write her up so fast it will make her wet her pants."

"Oh, no, don't do that; then we'll have two messes to clean up." Sherrie tried to ease the tension, but Bertha didn't think it was a bit funny.

"You need to get some backbone and stand up to these people like I do. Then things will get taken care of once and for all!"

Sherrie's frustration level was rising with Bertha's demands, and Bertha had only started her list. As Bertha went on and on, Sherrie listened and didn't say a word. When Bertha finally came up for air, Sherrie politely informed her that most of her complaints could be brought up before the Association meeting on Thursday night and the group of residents in attendance could hash them out.

"I knew you'd weasel your way out of dealing with them, Sherrie. But, never fear, I'll be back in here next Monday or even sooner if things don't change. Mark my words!"

Sherrie let Bertha's barbs bounce off her shoulders and boomerang back into Bertha's lap, but Bertha never felt them. As she wheeled herself out the door, she had one more question, "What are you going to do about Oscar's dandruff problem? It's getting worse. It could easily fall in the green bean casserole at the potluck, and if that happens, then I might as well just die."

CHAPTER FOUR

Sarah's First Visit

"There's life in the old dame yet!"
—Donald Marquis

Maria and Cat were up early, had the morning's routines taken care of, and the coffee brewing, and they were watching the clock for Sarah's arrival. When she didn't show up by 10:00 a.m., Maria was irritated.

"Why can't people be on time? They always have excuses; I wonder what Sarah's will be."

Maria had almost given up when Sarah knocked at 10:17. "Finally!" Maria breathed in relief, even though with her poor eyesight, she couldn't be sure of the exact time.

Cat let her in, and the reasons began. "Oh girls, I know I am late, but I was in a bad way last night. I couldn't sleep and the more I tried, the more wide awake I was, and then I had hot flashes like you wouldn't believe." Sarah fanned herself with both her hands.

"Hot flashes?" Maria injected quickly, as she was showing Sarah to a seat on the couch at the same time.

"Isn't that something at my age! But, my doctor said I will flash 'til I'm under the sod. Well, to make a long story short, the sun was almost up when I finally went to sleep. And then, wouldn't you know it, I had a dream about prunes. You know what they say; 'you know you are really old when you dream about prunes!'"

"No, I've never heard that, but, so then, did you sleep in?" Maria wanted to know the real reason Sarah was late.

"I guess I did. The last time I looked at the clock, I think it said 5:30, but you never know with these eyes without glasses. You know, the eye doctor says I have macular degeneration in both eyes. But, anyway, the next time I looked at the clock, it said 9:30, so I really had to hurry to get down here on time."

Maria opened her mouth to say, "You weren't on time," but all she got out was "You were . . ." when Cat interrupted with, "You were wanting coffee, Sarah?"

"Oh yes, thank you. I need it to wake me up and get my motor running, but then I'll be higher than a kite all day. I don't dare drink it too late in the day or I'll start the whole process of not sleeping tonight all over again. Does that ever happen to you, Maria?"

"Surely does. I like to have my mochas every day, but before 4:00 o'clock, if at all possible, but my reason is the bladder problem. I hate to get up and down all night."

Sarah, of course, could relate to that as well, and she launched into an organ recital about her personal plumbing and other important parts. "I heard on television the other night that the only thing golden about *The Golden Years* is a person's urine!"

Meanwhile, Cat was waving the cannoli recipe in her mother's face and wanting to get on with the cooking segment. As soon as Sarah had finished her recitation about her lungs with the statement that "pneumonia is the old person's best friend," Maria stood up. "I don't mean to be rude and I hate to cut this conversation short, but I have a million and one things to do, such as go to the office and get a few things cleared up, so could we look at the cannoli recipe now?"

"Here I am, rattling on again, and I don't even like to talk. Now Bertha does, and you won't get into that office on a Monday morning until she gets through griping to Sherrie about some picky, little things that get under her skin. Yes, Maria, tell me about this cannoli and how you make it. It sounds Italian. Oh, are you Italian?"

Maria nodded. "Yes, both my parents were from Tuscany on the west coast."

"My goodness! What a coincidence! I am intrigued with Tuscany! In fact, one of my dear friends knew that and she gave me a calendar last Christmas with pictures of Tuscany. Oh, Maria, I can tell that you and I are going to get along famously. I'll have to show you the calendar. It is just beautiful and every month I can't wait to turn it over for the new picture. I'll go and get it right now! We'll do the cannolis another time." With that she hurried out of their apartment, and they let her go!

"She sure gets side-tracked, doesn't she, Cat?"

"Yeah, she does, but I can't help but like her. She is quite a character and has quite a flair for the dramatics. Do you think she'll come right back?"

Maria shrugged her shoulders. "I have no idea. I'll give her a few minutes and then I think we should both go to the office. I want you to be there this first time and make sure I get everything straight. Do you mind, Cat?"

"No, that's what I'm here for, and we might meet some interesting people."

"Mixed nuts!" They chimed in unison and hugged each other on the way to the office.

They saw no sign of Sarah again that morning in their apartment nor in the lobby, so they just assumed she'd gotten side-tracked or had taken a nap. She'd surely be out at 7:00 p.m. to gather the sections of the daily paper from the library, but when Maria and Cat returned from a short walk around 7:10 that evening, Sarah was nowhere to be seen.

Bertha was patrolling the lobby and community room and the two hallways on the main floor. "Have you seen Sarah this evening?" Maria felt sure that Bertha would have an answer, and of course, she did.

Bertha drew her small frame into a ramrod position in the wheelchair. She pursed her lips and nodded her head before answering. "All I know is she left at 5:00 o'clock and here it is after seven and those newspapers are still there! I will have to bring that up at The Association meeting because she is shirking her duties, and we thought we could count on her."

"Has it ever happened before? Maybe she has a good reason." Cat couldn't help but stick up for their new-found friend.

"Well, she went out with that old man again, if you can call that a good reason."

Now Maria was interested. "That old man. What man?"

"I don't know who he is, but she has gone out with him before. He doesn't live around here. He wears a black leather jacket. Can you imagine?"

"I suppose he drives a Harley Davidson, too." Cat didn't know if Bertha liked to be teased or not, and frankly, she didn't care.

Finally someone had mentioned something about which Bertha knew nothing. "I suppose his name could be Mr. Davidson; we've never been introduced, but I could care less about his name. It's those newspapers I'm worried about."

Maria wanted to suggest that Bertha just wheel in the library and collect them on her lap and not cause such a stir over a one-time incident, but already she knew that Bertha did not operate that way, so she kept out of it. She did wonder about the man in the black leather jacket, though. In fact, she wondered enough that she and Cat sat in the lobby waiting for Sarah to return until almost nine o'clock. Just when they had almost yawned themselves to sleep, they heard a rumble from outside, the lobby doors swung open, and in walked Sarah all alone. All of a sudden, Maria and Cat both wished they could crawl under the rug and hide until Sarah was safely tucked away for the night in her upstairs apartment.

Sarah spotted them immediately as they stood and tried to sneak off down past the library.

"My, you two are up late. This is even better than Motel 6 leaving the light on. Were you waiting up for me ?" She was still gushing at that late hour.

Cat jumped in immediately with an answer. "Oh, hi, Sarah, we didn't see you come in. No, we were just visiting and getting acquainted with other residents and lost track of time. Did your bridge club run late this evening?"

Maria glared at her daughter and whispered. "Don't ask a question; you'll get a long answer."

"Bridge? Oh no, I wasn't at bridge. I went out for Chinese food and then for a drive with an old friend of mine. He just got a new car and wanted to show it off. It's a white convertible, but it was too cold to put the top down other than to show me how easy it is to operate. He's a spry gentleman, but for me, it was so hard to get in and out of it—so low!"

"Convertibles are fun! Did you see my red one out in the parking lot? Mom agrees with you about the low-slung cars, don't you, Mom? Mom!" Maria was yawning and about to doze off standing up.

"Oh, yes, it hurts my back, but we like to take it to the coast in the summer." Maria's mood changed quickly with the memories of the drive up 101 and all the way to Seaside.

Sarah was launching into a discussion about how she didn't like the wind in her ears or on her neck when the elevator arrived for her lift-off to the second floor.

"Oh, to be seventy again," Sarah sighed, as she pulled up her skirt and shook her left leg.

CHAPTER FIVE

Millie

"Beautiful young people are accidents of nature,
but beautiful old people are works of art."
—Eleanor Roosevelt

The lobby was teaming with anxious residents around "mail time." The mailman had alerted the administrator who had admonished the residents to stay back out of the way and let the mailman do his job and fill the boxes before they produced their keys and pounced on their slots to retrieve their bills or solicitations. But it was the highlight of their day, and most were like eager little children at Christmas waiting for Santa, so they could tear into their packages or letters. Essie was peering through the blinds, hoping to be the first to spot the mail truck and beat out Bertha just once!

"Here he comes!" Essie announced with glee.

"Oh, it is not! It's a taxi. That's Millie, coming back from the eye doctor." Bertha corrected her.

Essie calmed down and continued to peek through the slats of the blinds. She still hoped to see him first.

The doors swung open when Millie pushed the button and she swooped in. "I can't see a thing; my eyes have been diluted!" She announced to the congregation in the lobby, as she squinted and tried to recognize someone—anyone! "Am I in the right place? Everything is so bright."

Bertha took over. "Where are your sunglasses? What kind of a doctor wouldn't give you some dark glasses to wear? I'd change doctors if I were you."

Cat, who thought it was chic and cool to wear her glasses on top of her head, piped up.

"They are on your head, Millie, and I see they are designer sunglasses."

"Well, of course they are. That's where I always used to have them in Hollywood—on my head. Every one did. Are you from Hollywood, dear? I don't believe I know you. Are you the new lady?" Millie continued to squint at Cat.

"No, my mom Maria is the new lady. I'm just visiting. I have a home in Hillsboro."

Millie had latched onto Cat's arm for support. "Oh yes, I remember now. But you should move in here, too. It would be nice to have some young blood." She swept her arm over the lobby. "You see, dear, these are all old people!"

Cat was none too pleased with the invitation but cajoled Millie by saying, "Except for you!"

Millie felt like she was back performing and receiving a standing ovation. She thrived on the accolades and reveled in applause and compliments. In fact, she bowed and thanked Cat, as if she was coming back for an encore.

"You know, Sarah is always talking about her beautiful legs—her gams, as she calls them, and they're nice, I suppose, but look at me! Do you think I am still beautiful, dear? Now, look at my neck. See, it's not a turkey neck. I exercise it every morning and every night, and look at my cheeks. In fact, just touch them and see how soft they are and my face is not jowly like some around here. I eat right, too, and once a week, I have my cleansing cocktail of hot prune juice. Now, look at this lady ambling toward us. Just look at those jowls and that sagging neck." Millie's eyesight was coming back.

"That's my mom," Cat said, "and to me she is beautiful." Cat tried not to be offended. She'd been around "Hollywood" people before when she was married to Brock, a script writer for *The Young and the Restless*. The most beautiful people were often the most insecure people and needed to be praised and admired just to get through the day. That's why she was through with Brock. It just wasn't in her any more to hear all that talk about the beautiful people and lavish it on as thick as strawberry preserves day after boring day.

"Oh, I am so sorry. She is beautiful in her own way. Hello, Maria, Cat was just telling me how beautiful you are." Millie knew how to polish the apple, too.

Maria put her off. "Oh sure, but she's prejudiced. Has the mail come? No? Well, let's go, Cat. I need a mocha." She marched toward the door. "Come on, Cat," she urged.

"Some day soon I'll have to tell you about my career and my new plan," Millie hollered over the din of the over-anxious residents still waiting for the mailman.

"*You* need a mocha? Wow! So do I. See you, Millie," and they left her smoothing her neck and pouting. She loved to pout for attention, plus she thought it made her lips more sensuous and more pliable. Her lipstick was up higher than the actual lip to give a roundness and a fullness, she thought, but actually it looked smudged and messy. Nobody told her, because it did give her character. No one could say she had withered lips!

Millie had been vague about her acting career from the day she moved in a few months ago. Now and then she'd mention some obscure name of an actor or actress that had a bit part in an old movie, but never anyone that the residents could easily recognize. Sarah had wondered how she ended up at Pear Blossom Plaza in a HUD facility, and so one day she had just come right out and asked her. Millie's answer was shocking! "I am a charter member of Gambler's Anonymous. Lost it all, even my good name—Millicent Monroe—no relation to Marilyn, I might add. Now I am just plain, old Millie. It was fun while it lasted, but it's over, and now I want to move on and open a boutique right here. I am sick of our so-called garage sales! How can we have a garage sale? We don't even have a garage!"

CHAPTER SIX

The Shopping Trip

Cannoli: *A pastry roll with a creamy, sweet filling.*
Cannelloni: *Large tubes of pasta stuffed with meat or cheese and baked in a tomato or cheese sauce.*

While Maria waited out in front on the bench, Cat walked through the parking lot to the visitor spot where her car was parked. The sun was warm for a February afternoon, and, if she'd been by herself, Cat would have driven with the top down. Maybe when I go home, she thought, as she backed out and pulled around in front of the "home."

"Oh shoot, here comes the mailman now," Maria grumbled as she lowered her short, squat body into the bucket seat. "Let's go; we're in his spot, I think."

"Get that seat belt on, and we will." Cat was a stickler about that law.

"Can't you just slowly ease on out of his way and help me snap it in place at the same time? I can't find the hole. You know Bertha is watching and she'll write you up if you're in his spot."

"Yep, here we go, Mom. You're all hooked up. Let's roar on out of here," and she literally did that. "I need a break from those women. I think I'll have a triple shot of caffeine."

"So, you see how it is already. What chance do I have here? Do you think I'll make it, Cat? Now, I really am serious; do you think I can handle it?"

"Oh, I know you, Mom, and you will do just fine. Just pick out the nuts you like and leave the rest in the can. Ha. Ha. Little joke there, huh Mom?"

"Yeah, very little. But, I guess you are right. I'll just have to find a way to fit in. Which reminds me . . . I've been thinking about the potluck."

"Oh yes, the one thing you were never going to attend."

"Cat, now come on and hear me out. I've been thinking that since the sign-up sheet says 'we need more meat dishes,' maybe I should make cannelloni instead of cannoli."

"Whoop dee doo! I think you should, by all means, Mom. If nothing else, it will confuse everyone. If anyone looked it up in the dictionary, as Sarah suggested, then they are all primed for a pastry," Cat loved this idea and was glad she was staying for her mom's one and only potluck. She ran a red light, just thinking about it and anticipating the confusion.

Maria grabbed onto Cat's right arm. "Slow down; do you want to get a ticket like Jillian did? One of those cameras caught her, and she got the speeding ticket in the mail."

"Jillian always drives too fast, and so does Michael." Cat had ridden with her brother enough times in the Portland area to know he has a lead-foot. "But let's get back to the menu. Cannelloni will cost a lot more to make, but it is more sensible, and someday you could take the cannoli to the Saturday morning Koffee Klatch, and wow them at that, too."

"Possibly, if I go. Well, okay, if you'll help me make the dish for the potluck, then I'll go ahead and get the ingredients today, if you'll take me to the supermarket. Remember, we saw an Albertsons just up the street the other day." Maria was so excited that she forgot about her mocha.

Cat had not. "First things first, Mom. Here's the mocha stand," and she swung into the parking lot and up to the window. "Mom wants a 16 ounce iced mocha with . . ."

Maria shook her head. "No, I don't; I'm changing my ways. Tell that girl I want a 20 ounce Rogue River Rumble with two shots! I don't know what the heck it is, but I feel like living dangerously."

A few sips and a few blocks later, Maria and Cat, with their iced drinks firmly ensconced in the cup holders of the shopping cart, roamed the aisles of the supermarket in search of the cannelloni ingredients. Maria pulled out the recipe she'd tucked into her purse just in case Cat would agree to her already cemented-in-stone decision. Cat read off the necessary items to her mother as they scanned the shelves for Maria's favorite canned tomatoes and the extra lean hamburger, spiced up with a bit of Italian seasoned sausage. She insisted on making the meat department their last stop before the check-out line to insure that the meat was fresh.

Maria was the designated cart-pusher. "It gives me support," she insisted, and she pushed the cart into aisle Number 2, not noticing that it read, "12 items or less." Just up ahead of her was Winnie, tapping on the floor with her cane, as the clerk rang up her 11 items, most of which were bottles of red wine. Winnie scanned Maria's cart quickly.

"You have 13 items; you don't belong here." Winnie glared at Maria over her half-glasses. "Oh, it's you, the new lady. Well, what should I expect? You don't know your way around this town yet."

"No, that's not it. My mother knows how to shop—boy, can she ever shop! But she can't see the signs too well any more. I think you owe her an apology." Cat maybe didn't always agree with her mother's ideas or like her caustic attitudes, but she would defend her nevertheless to her dying day when someone else treated her like dirt!

"I don't do apologies, especially when there is nothing to apologize for," and with that, Winnie stomped out with her cane.

"Of all the nerve, treating you like that," Cat hissed, with venom on her breath.

"Oh well, Cat, just consider the source. I just wonder how much longer I am going to be called *The New Lady*."

Maria apologized to the check-out gal for having one-too-many items in her cart, but the clerk just brushed it off. "No big deal. By the way, do you know that woman who bawled you out? She comes in here almost every day for weeks on end, and then, all of a sudden, we don't see her for awhile, and when we asked her where she's been, she's very mysterious. We aren't trying to be nosy; we just hope she hasn't been sick, but she always says she's been out of town on important business."

Maria rolled her eyes and handed the clerk her check. "I'm afraid I *am* getting to know her; she lives just 3 doors down from me at Pear Blossom Plaza. I just moved in over the weekend from Roseburg. See, I haven't even had time to get the new address on my checks."

"Welcome to Middleford. My name is Kristin, and I see your name is Maria. What a delightful name! I hope you will shop here often and I can wait on you again, and good luck in your new home."

Maria looked around for Cat, who had disappeared. She saw her right behind her placing a can on the counter to be scanned.

"What's that? Did I forget something for the recipe?" Maria started fumbling in her purse for some money, but Cat waved her off.

"This is my treat, Mom. Mixed nuts!" Cat winked at her mother.

Upon arriving back at the home, Maria instructed Cat to set the groceries out in front, and she would get the grocery cart from the Community Room closet to transport the bags to her apartment. But the cart was gone. Bertha had the answer. "The new lady has it."

When Maria told her that *she* was the new lady, Bertha's reply was, "Not any more."

CHAPTER SEVEN

The Bird Lady

"You cannot fly like an eagle
with the wings of a wren."
—William Hudson

"Crystal chandeliers, linen table cloths, a rosebud on the table—in your dreams, Granny. You're not going to the Manor; you're going to the Home. I've been there making a delivery and the Manor is too good for you!" Billy continued his tirade as he shoved his grandma into the front seat of his old, brown Chevy, cinched the seat belt around her thin waist, and secured the locks, just in case she'd try the great escape.

"You're not rich enough to live at the Manor. You're so stupid! Giving all that money to your church!"

Blanche covered her face with her hands and sobbed, so she missed the good-bye waves and tears of her neighbor Martha across the street.

"Oh, shut up!" Billy hit the gas pedal hard and roared away from the curb. He saw Martha and wanted to make an obscene gesture, but why bother? She was just an old lady, too, and he had little time for them.

"Will you shut up?" He yelled at her again as Grandma continued to cry.

"I'll never see my home again; I just know it," she blurted out between sobs, as she fumbled for a tissue in her sweater pocket. She was tiny like a little bird, and the second-hand sweater from Goodwill could have wrapped around her twice.

"So what? You'll have a roof over your old, gray head and some grub a couple times a day. What more do you want? And besides, I have power of attorney, so I can do whatever I want with your house!" Billy's bragging exuded hatred.

"I don't know why I ever agreed to that. I'm not even dead yet; Why are you taking it away from me?"

"You're givin' it to me because I'm your favorite." Billy laughed loudly and the gap between his two front teeth looked more like the Grand Canyon than ever before, Blanche noticed, as she turned to stare at her grandson. She'd known him intimately for all of his 21 years, had changed his diapers and helped rear him when his parents got divorced, but this was a Billy she didn't recognize or even want to know.

She couldn't afford to live in her house any more. The taxes and heating bill had drained her bank account in November, and in December she had just hung on by her fingernails until Beau found this place for her in one of his more kindly moods. She suspected that both Beau and Billy were mixed up in the world of drugs. They both flashed money around at times and it was during those times that they treated her half-way decently, and then other times, like right now, when they were looking for a hand-out, they were as mean as feral cats. In fact, Billy was downright abusive. He'd slapped her around several times.

Thank goodness, it was a short ride to Pear Blossom Plaza. He drove so fast, he nearly hit a dog, and he passed a school bus with its lights flashing. All of a sudden, the tan apartment building was in sight, and Billy careened into the parking lot, left the motor running, and tore around to her side of the car.

"Get out!" Billy jerked the door open. He ran to the back of the car and threw up the trunk. The only belongings that Billy had room for were in three, big, black plastic garbage bags, and he threw those on the sidewalk. Her other son, Beau, would bring the furniture.

Blanche made it to the sidewalk just as Billy roared off. "Have a nice life," he muttered as he left his grandma standing there with tears pouring down her cheeks.

Just like when Maria moved in, Bertha and Antonio were stationed to greet the new lady. They were outside this time in the sunshine and were privy to all that had gone on as Blanche arrived. Antonio went to get the grocery cart to help her move in. Bertha, meanwhile, produced some tissues from her apron pocket and offered them to the new lady. Blanche wavered and staggered to the bench where she sat down hard, sobbing uncontrollably.

"Who in the world was that?" Bertha quizzed her. "Oh, try to get yourself together before you go in to meet your neighbors," Bertha continued impatiently.

Soon Antonio appeared with the grocery cart and helped Blanche load up the garbage bags. Of course, Bertha wondered what was in the bags, but for once, she had the good sense to keep her mouth shut and not ask. Antonio summoned Sherrie from the office to come and help get "the poor woman out front" calmed down and show her to her apartment. Like with Maria, other family members had viewed the apartments and made the arrangements, so it was all foreign territory—new faces, new walls to stare at, and new feelings with which to deal.

Giving up so much and finding so little. *Downsizing,* the senior citizen magazines and newspapers called it. *Cramped into a little box* was more like it. Complain or accept it. Adapt or fall apart.

At least Maria had a supportive family. Michael was across town, and Cat lived a few hours up north, so she didn't feel like she was just dumped off, whereas Blanche literally was. Like a bird pushed out of the nest to try her own wings, Blanche had landed at Pear Blossom.

Beau wasn't much more dependable than Billy. He had stored her *junk,* as he called it—furniture, dishes, pictures, and mementoes in a storage unit on Barnett. It was just down the hill, but Blanche was scared to try to retrieve her possessions on her own. If he'd only bring the big furniture, maybe she could find a way to get the rest of her belongings to her apartment, and, in the days and weeks to come, that's just what she did. The shopping cart would disappear for hours at a time only to reappear with Blanche pushing it through the parking lot and into the lobby. She kept to herself and although the residents knew her name was Blanche, they called her *The Bird Woman.* Her little spindly legs, a beak of a nose, and her twittering ways reminded them of a little wren on a wire.

Bertha didn't think the nickname was at all funny or polite. "She has a respectable name, you know, and she should be called by that."

"Here comes *The Bird Woman,*" was often heard, but no one admitted to calling her that to her face, and, in fact, they politely addressed her as Blanche.

On her first day, Blanche failed to return the shopping cart in a timely fashion, not yet knowing the rules nor that the enforcer, Bertha, ruled the place with an iron hand, and so when Bertha informed Maria and Cat upon their return from shopping that Maria was no longer *The New Lady,* she also stated that the newest *New Lady* had the cart, "and she's had it for an inordinate amount of time, I might add." Bertha proceeded to tell Maria and Cat all that had gone on out in front. "I was an eye witness!" Bertha announced proudly.

She went on to say, "We may have to handle her with gloves on for awhile. I think she's a victim of elderly abuse; I saw bruises, but far be it from me to get involved in that! That fellow that dropped her off—I mean literally dumped her out—should be shot! No wonder she's the emotional type, and a little bit of a scrawny thing, too. Antonio and Sherrie would have had to carry her in if she wouldn't have had the grocery cart to lean on. You missed a lot while you were out today."

Just then Cat returned from carrying the bags of groceries to the apartment. "You missed a lot, Mom, while we were out."

"I just heard that from Bertha," Mom replied.

Cat had more to report. "Well, I'll bet she didn't know that the calendar of Tuscany was shoved under the door, and on the door handle was another bag of Valentines candy, and the most interesting thing of all happened on the bulletin board. Your name was totally crossed off for Friday's potluck!"

"What? Who would do such a thing?" Maria couldn't believe her ears and hurried to see for herself. "I can't see it too well, but there is a heavy, black line through my name, alright. Of all the nerve! Just because I changed the menu item from cannoli to cannelloni doesn't mean I am not going, and remember, I had you erase that and change it. I just can't imagine who would do that!" Maria was huffing and puffing her way to the apartment. "I hardly even know anybody here yet!" She continued to fret.

"It must be a mistake," Cat tried to reassure her that nobody disliked her that much.

"I'll get a pen and go write your name and your dish in on another line." She left her mother wondering if she should even bother to cook and to attend.

Winnie was stomping down the hallway when Cat opened the door of the apartment She stopped for a moment, lifted her cane in the air and unscrewed the top portion of the walking stick. She pulled a black cord and attached was a small, silver flask which slid from her cane. Winnie quickly brought it to her lips and shot down a swallow. Then, looking behind her, she saw Cat was watching. "What are you looking at?" She hissed at Cat, who was glancing at her watch.

Thinking that two could play this game, Cat hissed back, "Oh, I was just thinking that it's five o'clock somewhere, but not here; it's only four thirty."

CHAPTER EIGHT

Josie Winters

"And a little child shall lead them."
                                    —Isaiah

Through the eyes of the elderly, things look different. Colors have faded, writing has blurred. Meals taste bland or are too spicy. Time goes so slowly or moves too fast.

Voices sound mumbled to their ears, or they don't sound at all. They are put in categories:

"He's stone deaf; she can't see a thing; Oh, you mean the one with the grey hair? She's the one who lost her husband; he's lost his marbles!" And on and on . . .

Josie Winters was not a child when she began volunteering at Pear Blossom last year, but the residents saw the seventeen-year-old girl through the eyes of their own youth. With long, blonde hair, a flawless, clear complexion, and a smile that could dazzle the dimmest vision, Josie wound herself around the hearts of the residents like an ivy plant winds around an arbor. Those that had never even liked children were enamored with her beauty, but even more so with her gentle, loving heart. She cared for each one of them, and they could feel it. They were astounded that one so young would even pay any attention to them, but she thought of each one, not as just one who had been put out to pasture, but as a grandparent that she had never had. Her grandparents were all elderly when she was just a baby, and before she could even say their names, they had gone to their final reward. Oh, sure she had favorites at Pear Blossom, but she knew what favoritism was like at school, and her heart broke for those who were put down and made fun of. Some were laughed at because they had to ride the school bus instead of having their own car; others were taunted because of the way they dressed or because they were too "prissy" and wouldn't go out and have some "real" fun.

The ultimate put-downs were made toward Josie's 6 year-old brother who had Down Syndrome. If they had only looked beyond Jake's physical body or through his round, thick glasses to the window of his soul, they would have seen his loving heart. Josie defended Jake as best she could, but she didn't always hear the name-calling or the laughter behind his back. When she did, it broke her heart, and she vowed she would never make fun of another human being.

Josie had played the organ at Pear Blossom a few times and knew some of the regulars, but only by sight and not by name. The last time she played, one lady had cried the whole time.

"Didn't you like my songs? I tried to play what I thought you'd like. I'm so sorry." Josie felt like she had failed in some way, but she didn't know what she had done.

The lady was Essie. "Oh, they just broke my heart; they reminded me of my home, and all the dead people in my family. And then Bertha wanted *My Old Kentucky Home,* and that's where I'm from! Kentucky!" Essie burst into tears again.

"How about if I play one more song just for you before I go home tonight?" Josie tried to soothe Essie's broken heart. "What would you like to hear?"

"*I'm Looking Over a Four-Leaf Clover* is one of my favorites," Essie said, as she wiped her eyes.

Josie didn't know that one, but she found it in the songbook and did the best she could and promised to learn it by the next Wednesday—"Just for you, Essie. Is that what I heard someone call you?"

"Yes, bless you, child. You brought a song to my heart and joy to my soul. Oh say, do you know *Cool Waters* or *Tumbling Tumbleweeds?* Those are my two favorite cowboy ones."

Josie had never heard of them. The only country music she liked at all was by Brooks and Dunn, but she assured Essie she'd try to learn those two for the next Wednesday gathering. She'd been practicing some Bobby Vinton tunes that her mother had found and some love songs for Valentines Day, but now Josie wondered if they would "break someone's heart."

*   *   *

Wednesday

It had been a big day at Pear Blossom. Sarah got a manicure and a pedicure, even though she couldn't afford either one, Millie had her eyebrows and her chin waxed, Gayle gave her dog a bath, the twins washed their hair with some new dandruff shampoo that Sherrie recommended, and Maria found a beautician, although she couldn't get in until Thursday afternoon. All of this took place on Wednesday—the sing-along night,—because the rumor was that Josie was bringing a special guest. A special guest could be anyone, and their imaginations ran wild.

Sarah thought maybe Josie was bringing her boy friend, Millie was sure it must be a famous musician coming to help her entertain, and Bertha was positive that it was a member of Josie's church choir. Maria had no idea, as she'd never heard of Josie. She knew there was a *Josie and the Pussycats,* "but wasn't that a movie?" she asked Cat.

Josie and her *assistant*, as she liked to call her brother Jake, to bolster his ego, arrived early on Wednesday evening, and she was all ready playing some tunes when the residents started streaming in. Jake was seated on the organ bench beside her, and when she nudged him, it was his job to turn the pages.

Maria and Cat were the first to arrive, as Maria made it a point to never be late for anything. Also she liked to sit in the first row and in the chair closest to the door, just in case *Mother Nature* decided to make an unexpected and urgent call. Of course, most of the residents clamored for that seat and for the same reason.

Sarah arrived and was happy to find an open seat next to Cat. She paused and hugged Maria first. "Oh, I'm so glad you two came; I was afraid you'd still be too busy in your apartment for a social gathering. But you wouldn't want to miss it; Josie is so talented and sweet! Sarah turned and glanced at Josie. "I wonder who that little boy is with her," she said, and looked at Maria, who shrugged her shoulders unknowingly.

"Sit here by me," Cat hugged Sarah, too. "It's nice to see you again. We were wondering too about the young child."

Just then the formidable Bertha wheeled in and parked on the end of the row next to Maria. Her wheelchair took up so much space that others couldn't get in from that end of the row and had to enter from the middle aisle.

"Who is that with Josie? Oh, my goodness! Look at him! He's a Mongoloid!" Bertha said much too loudly. Josie must have heard her because she held the note she was playing far longer that the 4 beats the music called for.

"Shhhhh," Maria tried to hush Bertha up. "You're too loud, plus Cat tells me now they are called *Down Syndrome*."

"Well, whatever he is, what is he doing here? I heard Josie was bringing a special guest, but I had no idea it would be a child and one like that!"

"He really is special!" Sarah tried to smooth things over, as the others came in and found their seats.

Josie stood up, right at seven p.m. and in a loud, clear voice that the most hearing-impaired ears could hear, she made an announcement.

"Hi, everyone. Tonight is a very special night. In two days it will be Valentine's Day and I know you probably want to hear some love songs, and also I brought someone special with me." She nudged Jake and whispered to him to stand up and take a bow. "I would like you all to meet my little brother Jake. He is my assistant tonight."

Jake grinned from ear to ear and waved and bowed several times. He clapped and waved until Josie nudged him again to be seated.

The evening went on delightfully with Josie playing a few tunes she had selected, and then she took requests from the audience. Most of the songs she knew fairly well or she was able to figure them out from the songbook. Jake turned the pages when she gave him his cue. When he began yawning and the residents began to run out of requests, Josie knew it was time to wind it up, and she stood and faced the group again.

"It's been fun for Jake and for me and I hope you all had a good time, too," she said. "I know Essie wants to hear *Cool Water,*" she said, as she found Essie in the crowd, "and then I hope you don't mind if we close with *Twinkle, Twinkle Little Star*. It's Jake's favorite song, and we sing it every night before he goes to bed. Let's all clap for Jake to sing."

"Oh, brother!" Bertha muttered to herself, but loudly enough that Maria heard her.

"Yes, it is her brother. Let's sing with him when he starts," Maria gently poked Berth in the ribs with her elbow, and Jake stood and smiled and began after Josie had finished.

Jake didn't need any assistance from Maria or anyone else. His voice was loud and clear as a bell, and he looked heavenward and pointed to the sky. One almost felt as if the the stars were twinkling through the ceiling of the Community Room, and several residents had tears in their eyes. Essie, who had remained dry-eyed throughout the love songs, pulled a Kleenex from her new box of tissues that she had bought at the Grocery Outlet especially for tonight's sing-a-long.

When Jake had hit the final note and bowed several times, Josie went to Essie and gave her a big hug. "Oh, it was soooo beautiful. Just like my little boy used to sing it." Essie sobbed and whispered into Josie's ear. "He was a Down Syndrome little boy, too."

"Let's talk some time soon, Essie." Josie hugged her again. "I have to get Jake home, but I'll come back and see you, maybe next week, okay?"

Essie clung to Josie for dear life. "Oh, please do come. It would be wonderful."

Maria and Sarah and several others thanked Josie and Jake, and Cat gave Jake a high-five. "Good job, Jake. I can tell you like to sing."

Jake hugged Cat. "I like you," he said.

"I like you, too. I hope you come again with Josie. I don't live here, but I might see you again."

Jake was pulling on his sister's sweatshirt and pointing to Cat. "Guess what? She likes me!"

"We all do!" Sarah had to get in on the lovefest.

Bertha looked at the group with disdain and wheeled out the door. "What is this place coming to?" She shook her head and wheeled over near the door of the library.

"I tell you true, it was a wonderful evening!" Sarah had appointed herself a committee of one to escort Josie and Jake to the front door. "We all loved it!"

"Not the lady in the wheelchair." Josie had observed her disgust.

"Oh, don't take it personally; She doesn't like anyone. She doesn't even like herself."

CHAPTER NINE

Betty and the Bra

"An advanced old woman
is uncontrollable by
any earthly force."
—Dorothy Sayers

Elected by the Association, approved by the administrator, and applauded by the other residents, Betty Hollis was the Activities Director at Pear Blossom Plaza. She resided right next door to Maria, and when the two met, the first words out of Betty's mouth were, "It is so nice to hear flushing going on just on the other side of the wall. I've really missed that, especially in the mornings, since the old lady died in her bed there, and they had to clean and paint the place."

"A cheery thought," Maria answered back, not knowing that she was sleeping in a dead person's bedroom. "How long has it been empty?" Maria queried Betty.

"Several weeks, actually. It took the relatives awhile to dispose of things, and then Tony had to do the renovations. They were too cheap around here to get him any assistance. Lord knows, I offered to help, but oh no, it had to be an employee. He would even come on his days off, just to speed things up so you could move in."

"I'm beholden to him," Maria said, "Just so it's clean."

"Oh, my yes! The exterminators were here, and the inspectors were here twice."

Maria frowned. "Exterminators? Were there mice or just bugs?"

"I think it is just the government's policy and it doesn't mean anything bad was living in your apartment. You know how these government watchdogs are."

"Yeah, Bertha should work for them, or maybe she does?" Maria was being facetious, but not one hundred per cent.

Betty was a clean and neat person herself, and her apartment was impeccable. She was not the Gestapo, though, nor did she run to Sherrie every time something was awry. Bertha had turned her in a couple times, though, for not meeting up to standards.

Once Bertha complained that she did not think there were enough activities and the residents were bored, and then the new game table was too high and Bertha couldn't reach it from her wheelchair without hurting her neck. Sherrie advised her to sit on some cushions and that seemed to placate Bertha for the time being.

"I'm just on pins and needles around here," Betty confided to Maria. "Why, at my age, do I have to worry about doing something wrong like a little kid? Now, today it is Thursday, the day before the potluck, and I think the kitchen in the Community Room needs cleaning, and I am happy to do it, but I suppose Bertha will find fault," Betty said in her deep, gravely voice from years of cigarette smoking.

Maria was quick to jump on Betty's bandwagon. "Well, if she doesn't like it, then next time she can do it herself. We would help you, but today is the day I go for my hair cut and set, and Cat has to drive me. I need a perm, but will have to wait until next week for that."

"I need a perm, too, in the worst way," Betty said, as she shook her white, dust mop of a hairdo. "I wish we could get someone to come here and do our hair. It would be a lot easier for those who don't drive. Well, I'm off to the kitchen. Wish me luck." She waved a cleaning rag at Maria and Cat. She wouldn't have minded their help, she guessed, but quite frankly, she liked to do it herself quietly and quickly without the advice of others.

The kitchen in the Community Room was not used daily because the residents had their own kitchens and fixed their own meals. Sometimes on Game Nights someone would make daiquiris and use the blender and always on Saturday mornings for the Koffee Klatch the coffee pots were brewing. The monthly potluck was the big attraction and for that the kitchen was used for serving and cleanup. Also a resident could reserve the room for a special family gathering or party, if nothing else was scheduled for that particular day. So, like any other kitchen, it got dirty, and needed *deep cleaning*, as Betty called it, and that was more than just a swipe of the dishrag over the countertops or a quick mop of the floor.

"What is that smell?" Winnie wondered aloud to Sarah, as they encountered each other in front of the elevator shortly after Betty had begun her assault on the cupboards.

"Well, it smells like some kind of a strong cleaning solution and it's coming from the kitchen. I hope I'm not allergic to it. My allergies, you know, are so . . . so diversified."

Sarah had to search for just the right descriptive word, so Winnie could fully appreciate her malady. She and Winnie did not get along, so it was unusual for Sarah to be so generous with her information.

They both peered into the kitchen, neither one wanting to enter it all the way until they could see what was going on.

"Oh, it's Betty. Hi Betty," Sarah was thrilled to see her. She and Betty saw eye to eye on things, and, in fact, Betty had secretly named Sarah as her assistant activity director. Mostly, Sarah was just a consultant because she had such good ideas for entertainment, and then she left it up to Betty and Gayle to act on and carry out her ideas.

They made a good team, but Betty hadn't asked Sarah to help clean. She knew of Sarah's allergies and how she wanted to keep her nails nice at all times.

Betty waved and said, "I'm rippin' right along here. It's not as dirty as I thought it would be. In fact, I'm almost done." She didn't want Winnie coming in and bothering her, so she pretended to be just finishing up. But Winnie had stomped into the kitchen and was rubbing her hands over the counter underneath the kitchen window. She pointed to a spot with her cane.

"There's some sticky stuff here that you missed, Betty."

"I didn't *miss* it; that is my last area to clean up!" Betty was grinding her teeth and biting her tongue and wanting a cigarette.

"Come on, Winnie. Let's go and wait for the mailman and let her finish up." Sarah's diplomacy nearly killed her, but she knew Betty needed some space, and she needed to get away from the strong odor of Lysol.

What she didn't know was what Betty had found in one of the cupboards. Nestled right next to the extra can of coffee and the filters was a woman's bra. Betty couldn't believe her eyes as she pulled the large, beige item of lingerie from the kitchen cupboard. What is that doing there? she wondered, as she examined it thoroughly. It appeared to be brand new and was neatly folded just as if it had come out of a box in the store. She had heard voices, so quickly shoved it into the large pocket of her apron. Not knowing what to do with it, she took it back to her apartment when she finished cleaning and worried over it all afternoon, like a cat worries over a mouse. She'd leave it and come back to it, touch it, hold it up and look at it, and lay it back down. She wished it *was* a mouse and would just run into a corner and hide.

Around 5:00 p.m., she decided that Cat and Maria must be back from the hair appointment, so she gingerly tapped on Maria's door. Cat ushered her in to where Maria was seated on the couch.

"Hi there, Betty. We finally got home. It took that hairdresser a long time."

"Your hair looks so pretty. Did you like the lady who did it?" Betty was searching for a new salon, so hoped Maria had some suggestions.

Maria stalled with her answer. "Actually, it was . . . okay. Well, actually, a man did it. I had no choice because the lady I had booked with was out with the flu, so this fellow was taking her appointments. I rather liked him, though, and I never thought I would say that about a male hair stylist."

"I've never been to one, but I have nothing against them; as long as they go to beauty school and are trained, what's the difference?" Betty was accepting of the trends of the 21st century. "Not to change the subject . . . but I will. I have been dying to show you what I found in the Community Room cupboards in the kitchen," and she pulled the bra out of her pocket and unfurled it like a flag.

"Well, for evermore. What in the world? Well, Betty, who would put that in the kitchen cupboard?" Maria was as taken aback as Betty, and Cat wasn't far behind.

"Look at the size of it!" Maria gasped, as Betty held it out at arm's length. "Who around here is that big? Just look at those cups!"

"We do have a couple of biggies, but even so, I don't know why they would put it in the kitchen cupboards." Betty was still incredulous of her morning's discovery.

"Yeah, if mine were that big I would want to hide them in my bottom drawer of my dresser! And mine are big enough, but not that big!" Maria laughed as Betty twirled it around in her living room.

Betty finally sat down and folded up the bra. "I guess I will have to put it in the lost and found, but even though it isn't mine, it is a little embarrassing and think of the gossip."

"Oh, well, it will give them all something new to chew on. Of course, once Bertha finds out about it, she'll investigate it. See, Betty, I've only been here a few days, but I am catching on fast, don't you think?"

Betty agreed, "Yes, she's the one to watch out for and Winnie is another one. She came in while I was cleaning and had a tizzy over a sticky spot on the counter."

Cat, who'd been sitting quietly on the sidelines, shook her head. "All these little trivial things get blown up way out of proportion around here. I guess some people just have nothing better to do than horn in on other people's business."

Maria and Betty both agreed that what Cat had observed and just stated was absolutely true; the little confines of an apartment and the residents' problems were sometimes all that was left to a person's life and they weren't able to physically or emotionally look beyond or see how their actions affected others. Little things became enormous.

"Cat, remember what I have always told you, 'Just consider the source.'"

"And bear with us," Betty added. "Oh, by the way, are you coming to the Association meeting tonight? I'd better get out of here so you can get ready."

"No, I don't think so. Not this time. Cat will be leaving in a few days and I want to spend as much time together with her as I can. Maybe next time, okay?" Maria hoped she wouldn't offend Betty by not showing up. "You do understand, don't you?"

Betty was coughing and sputtering and trying not to cry. "Yes, probably more than you will ever know! You are so lucky to have a daughter like Cat. Someday I'll tell you about my daughter, but for now, I must go put the bra away and get ready for the meeting," and with that Betty walked out the door leaving question marks dangling in the air.

*   *   *

Late that night after the meeting had dissolved into Bertha being right about the garden box situation and Blanche's use of the grocery cart, and Millie's request again for a Jacuzzi had been rebuffed one more time, Betty knew she still had to deal with the bra. Like an albatross hanging around her neck or a nagging in the pit of her stomach, the beige bra had been in the back of her mind all through the meeting, and now as it hung from the antennae of her television, she had an idea. Opening the door of her apartment, she stealthily looked up and down the hallway and listened for any activity in the lobby or the library. Often the television would be humming away, and Essie would be snoring on the couch along with Jay Leno and his guests. But tonight all was quiet.

Betty tiptoed past Maria's apartment and approached the first bulletin board that was reserved for notices of articles for sale, rides available, death notices, and lost and found items. First, Betty attached with a thumbtack a small recipe card to the bulletin board, which stated that a bra had been found. Right next to it, with two more thumbtacks, Betty pinned the bra to the bulletin board. She moved it several times—first hanging it vertically, but it was so long that it hung way down below the wood, so then she stretched it out horizontally. That was even more dramatic and filled in the empty spots of the board. As she stood back to admire it and to revel in her mischievous act, she heard a door opening.

It was Cat. Betty put her finger to her lips and tapped them several times, so Cat would know she wanted silence. Then she motioned for Cat to come over by the bulletin board.

"Look what I did!" Betty whispered in glee.

Cat was in shock. "Have you been drinking from Winnie's flask?" She inquired of Betty in a hushed whisper and with a smirk on her face.

"No, but I did have a little sip of wine before and after the meeting. Well, actually I had several sips after the meeting. It helps me sleep, you know, after all the anxiety I had bottled up all day. By the way, what are you doing out and about? Is Maria all right?"

"Mom? Oh, she's snoring like a bulldozer. I just couldn't sleep, so thought I would take a walk. I have an idea for a new book, and it keeps buzzing around in my head."

Betty was interested, as she loved to read. "You could write about this place. There are certainly some brilliant character studies to build a story around. Oops, I ended that sentence with a preposition and that is a no-no." Betty was feeling her oats.

"We'll let it go this time, but back to the bra. Are you going to leave it there?"

Betty at that point had no intentions of taking it down, but after Cat and she parted and went back to their respective apartments, Betty began to wonder if maybe she should remove it. Nope. I'm going to leave it there and see what happens in the morning. Cat surely won't squeal on me, so nobody will be the wiser, and someone might just claim it.

Betty, for once, was in the catbird seat and enjoying the view and the hilarity.

*   *   *

Bertha and Essie were called by phone at 7:30 a.m. Friday morning to the side hallway to view the embarrassment. Winnie had observed the whole thing from a chair in the short recess of a doorway that opened out onto the side parking lot, and the eager anticipation of tattling on Betty had kept her awake the entire night. She wanted Bertha and Essie to see it before Sherrie arrived, and so the three of them convened in front of the bulletin board shortly after the summoning phone call from Winnie.

"That's the last straw for Betty. I will see that she is evicted!" Bertha vowed.

PEAR BLOSSOM PLAZA COMMUNITY BULLETIN BOARD

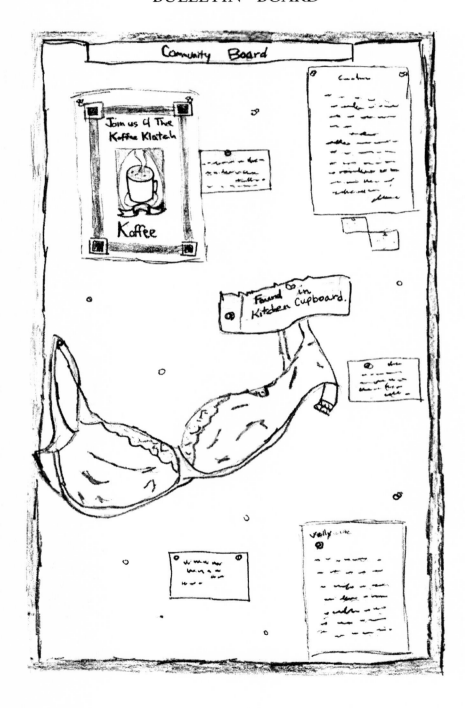

REVISED POTLUCK SCHEDULE
FRIDAY, FEBRUARY 14 6:00 P.M.

DO NOT SIGN UP TO BRING DESSERT; IT WILL BE PROVIDED

NAME	FOOD ITEM
1. Millie	Cheese curls
2. Sarah	Baked Chicken
3. Bertha	Garden Salad
4. Essie	Green Salad
5. Antonio and Tony	Chili and Cornbread
6. Winnie	Red or Green jello
7. Otis	Olives and Pickles
8. Oscar	Cake
9. B.K.	Relish tray
10. Maria & Cat	Cannelloni
11. Gayle	Green Bean Casserole
12. Pastor Paul	Rolls
13. Blanche	------------------
14. Carol and Dave	Baked Squash
15. Emily and Herb	Au Gratin Potatoes

REPEAT: DO NOT BRING ANY DESSERT. IT IS PROVIDED.

CHAPTER TEN

Valentine's Day

"I am so glad when it is time to celebrate this day
Because I have a grand excuse to give my heart away."
—James J. Metcalfe

A shroud of fog hung heavy over the golf course, wrapping itself over the shoulders and limbs of trees and covering the grass with sparkling diamonds. It was quiet and still—one of those mornings that waits in hushed silence for the rays of the sun to gently lift the covering and breathe new life into day.

That was outside, east of the patio and just across the creek, and was the view that Maria, Betty, and Winnie had from the first floor and others had from the second and third floors. They awakened each day to witness the changing seasons from their bedroom windows, while those on the west side had the cold, concrete parking lot and the office annex building to greet them each morning.

Inside Pear Blossom Plaza on that Valentine's Day, the activities began early. In fact, the exciting part of Betty's escapades carried over from the night before. While Betty slept, exhausted from the kitchen cleaning, the meeting, and her late-night antics, Bertha, Winnie, and Essie waited impatiently for Sherrie to arrive and open her office door. Cat, too, was worn out from thinking about the plot for her next novel, and then finding Betty hanging "cups" on the bulletin board.

Maria was up early, as usual, and she tiptoed around the kitchen, taking her 13 pills and making coffee. They had forgotten to take the meat out of the freezer for the cannelloni, so Maria was panic-stricken that it wouldn't thaw in time.

Out in the hallway, Cupid was busy hanging Valentines on certain doorknobs. He'd been up late into the night, as well, thinking about the right wording for his cards.

Cat drifted in and out of her dreams until suddenly she became fully awake and found her mother standing by the hide-a-bed with her hands on her hips.

Rubbing her eyes to try to get some semblance of alertness, Cat looked around to find her bearings. "Oh, my gosh, I was having an awful dream about my dog. I thought I heard her scratching at the door, and when I opened it, she had a noose around her neck; she isn't here, is she? Oh, my gosh, I know why I had that dream of something hanging," and she proceeded to tell her mother about Betty's decorations on the bulletin board.

Maria thought it was hilarious at first, but then sobered up. "There'll be trouble over that. Poor Betty! She will have to answer to 'you-know-who.' Now, get up! You have to help me. The meat is frozen solid, and I don't know what to do. I don't mean to trivialize Betty and the bra . . . or maybe I do, but I have my own troubles, you know."

Cat glanced at the clock. "Oh yes, it's the big day—cooking day." With that realization, she heaved herself out of bed and grabbed her mom around the waist and kissed her on the cheek. "Happy Valentine's Day, Mom. Do you think your new sweetie will give you some candy?"

"Caterina Maria Manchini, I do not have a sweetie! Now, help me!"

Cat, who was sooooo thankful she had shortened her name, took hold of her mother's hand and pulled her into the kitchen. "Look over at the tray by the wall, and you will see one of the greatest inventions of mankind—the microwave. Now, I know, you've told me time after time that you don't know how to use it other than to heat up water, so today I will give you a lesson on how to thaw hamburger—oops, I mean ground beef and the sausage. You will love it, and it will make life so much simpler for you."

"I'll try, but there is one other problem; I can't see to read the numbers or the lettering." Maria's reluctance to try new things had always held her back, but she had a legitimate reason for being fearful this time.

"Not to worry, Mom. Here, look at it closely. I have put bigger numbers on each pad that the Middleford Blind Association gave me—you know, like we put on your phone."

So, with lessons going on in Apartment 101, Bertha finally making her way into the office, and Tony rearranging the tables and chairs in the Community Room for the potluck, Valentine's Day was taking shape.

Sherrie had loved Valentine's Day all her life. Growing up, she had decorated the obligatory shoe box card holders in elementary school, danced the evening away in high school at the Valentine's dances with whomever she was dating that particular year, and then she met the love of her life in college. She and Randy had been married for three years now, and February 14th became more special with every passing year. Randy was the romantic type, and he always tried to outdo the previous year's celebrations.

This year Randy made the plans to go up to Roseburg for dinner and then drive over to Bandon on the coast on Saturday for the rest of the weekend. Sherrie had packed a bag late Thursday night, "enough for three days," he told her, but she had no idea where they were headed. She had been asked time and again to come back Friday night for the potluck, and as much as she hated to turn them down, a night in the Community Room with the same folks she'd seen all week, just didn't compare to a weekend away with Randy. Bertha's tirade this morning had hermetically sealed her decision to skip the potluck.

"Maybe next month," she told Bertha, just to placate her for the time being.

"Maybe next month we won't even be here." Bertha replied, which made no sense to Sherrie. Bertha had demanded Betty's eviction, but Sherrie had told her she had no grounds to kick her out. There was no place in the rules for bulletin board infractions. In fact, Sherrie had to stifle her laughter and applause for Betty's gusto. She suggested that she and Bertha go and view the heinous crime together, and, of course, Bertha was more than willing to show Sherrie the awful, "almost pornographic" desecration in the hallway.

However, to their amazement the bra was gone! Even the lost and found card looking for the bra's owner had been removed.

"Well, I guess that takes care of it," Sherrie said, breathing a sigh of relief.

"Not necessarily. Now I will have to investigate and see who removed it. Maybe Betty came to her senses or maybe someone stole it!" Bertha was not ready to let go of the matter so easily.

As they turned to go back toward the lobby together, Bertha spied a Valentine card and gift hanging from Maria's doorknob. "That's wrong, too. It specifically says in our booklet of rules that we are not to leave things on other people's doors. Look it up if you don't believe me."

Sherrie had to agree with Bertha that time. "Yes, you are correct, but since she is so new and it is Valentine's Day, we can't judge too harshly. We'll let it go this time."

"Well, someone else caused the infraction—not Maria. So that person should be punished. I wonder who it was that hung it there." Bertha's curiosity was killing her.

"Don't you dare look, Bertha. Come on. Let's go and have some coffee and settle down. It will soon be found and will disappear."

"No, I am going upstairs to check other doorknobs. Maybe that is not the only one," and with that, Bertha punched the elevator button, rolled in, and disappeared.

She made her rounds of the second and third floors, and she did discover one other Valentine. It was suspended from Millie's doorknob, and she hurried back downstairs to report it to Sherrie. Surprisingly, the office door was locked and a note hung in the glass window that stated that the office was closed for the rest of the day. Sherrie had gone home with a migraine. Bertha grunted and rolled down the west wing to her apartment.

"I wish I could be the administrator and then things would get taken care of properly around here," she said aloud, as she looked in her hand mirror. "But, oh no, you have to be young and beautiful to hold a position like that, not some withered up old paraplegic in a wheelchair." She tossed the mirror on the bed, hoping it would break. "Valentine's Day? Who cares?" she muttered to herself. "Maybe I won't even go to the potluck. They'll just have to get along without my garden salad."

*   *   *

Sarah had slept soundly for a change and had missed all the excitement. Being up on the second floor was a detriment in that way, but, in another way, she was often glad to escape the trivialities of goings-on in the lobby and the hallways. She thrived on fun things, but not on the gossip or Bertha's criticisms and intolerance of others.

When the ringing phone jolted her fully awake at 9:30 and she heard Maria's voice on the other end, she was happy to start the day with her new-found friend, and she came to life immediately.

"Oh, good morning, Maria . . . . No, you didn't awaken me; I've been up and dressed for hours. I'm in a bad way, you know, with these hot flashes again all night, and now I have a terrible itch on my left forefinger. I just don't know what it is. My friend had it too, and her dermatologist cleared it right up. You know, the friend who gave me the Tuscany calendar. I must phone her and get her doctor's name."

"Why did I call her?" Maria was mouthing to Cat, who didn't know if Maria had really forgotten why or if she was regretting dialing her number.

"That's too bad." Maria tried to drum up some sympathy. It paled in comparison to all her ailments, but she figured to Sarah it was just as worrisome as her own high cholesterol. "Say, I was just wondering if you'd like to come down and watch us make the cannelloni. Then you'd know first-hand what it is and how to make it. What do you think?"

"What a delightful invitation! Now, what time are you starting it? I have a couple pressing things to do right away." Sarah hoped to stall her, so she could at least get dressed and eat a bran muffin.

"How about eleven? Will that give you enough time to iron out things?" Maria was anxious to get the dish put together and refrigerated and move on to other things, but she could wait one more hour. That would give Cat ample time to get her shower and get the meat thawed.

"Perfect," Sarah had no idea what time it was, but agreed anyway. "I'll hurry and make my calls. Oh, my stars. Don't let me forget to cook the chicken!"

The hour flew by. Sarah stopped in the lobby on her way to Maria's just to see what was going on. It was fairly quiet for a Friday morning, but with it being a potluck day, Sarah figured the cooks were squirreled away, cooking their favorite dishes or dumping the cheese curls into a bowl. Even Bertha was nowhere to be seen or heard.

The Valentine was still hanging on Maria's doorknob with a curly red ribbon. Sarah left it so Maria could see it when she opened the door. She tapped and Cat let her in.

Cat's bright eyes spotted it swinging as the door opened. "Oh, look, Mom, your sweetie has been here all ready!"

"Maria, you didn't tell me you had a boy friend here. How nice! Do I know him?"

"Look what you've started, Cat. I don't have a *sweetie* or a *boyfriend* or whatever you want to call him." Maria was provoked, but curious at the same time and opened the envelope carefully. There was no name; it said, "FOR MY VALENTINE."

Cat spoke up, "We think it must be Antonio who has designs on her."

Sarah thought that either Maria knew him from the outside from before she moved in, or else she was a fast worker, but Maria assured her that she had never met the man until he greeted her at the front door on moving-in day.

"Are you going to read it, Mom?" Cat and Sarah were overly-anxious, especially to see who had tied it to the door.

If Maria had really thought it would be mushy or a private matter, she would have put it aside for later, but having no idea it would be so full of love, she asked Cat to read it aloud.

She could share all this nonsense, she thought.

"What a pretty card!" Cat held it up for all to see, and then she began to read.

VALENTINE WISHES

I offer you my grateful heart
And all my love today
And many are the wishes now
That I sincerely say.
I wish you all the happiness
That you could ever hold . . .
A silver dawn, a sky of blue,
And moments made of gold.
I wish you health and comfort
And a perfect peace of mind,
With melodies and memories
That leave all cares behind.
I wish you every blessing, dear,
That heaven can bestow.
And may your noble virtues and
Your charms forever grow,
And more than these I wish today
In every word and line
To cherish you forever as
My loving Valentine.
—Poem by James J. Metcalfe

Sarah had her hand over her heart, and tears had formed in the corners of her eyes. "I usually have such dry eyes and have to use drops, but those words would eliminate that medication! Nobody has ever sent *me* a card like that, and I was married for over 50 years."

Maria didn't know whether to laugh or cry. "So, is it from Antonio?" she queried Cat.

Cat frowned and put her forefinger under her nose and her thumb under her chin, so she could study and contemplate the question. "It doesn't really say. It is signed, 'With love. I will miss you.'"

"'Miss you?' I'm not going anywhere!" Maria was baffled.

"Maybe Antonio is going away. You know, that is a possibility. Did you think of that, Maria?" Sarah thought she had the solution.

"Or maybe it is not from Antonio. Maybe you have another admirer." Cat thought she had it solved.

Maria had another idea, but didn't offer it.

"Well, let's put it aside for now and get on with the recipe," Maria was in the cooking mood. "Cat, open the window. It sure has gotten warm in here, and the oven isn't even on yet."

The recipe came together with the three of them working in the little, cramped kitchen.

Somehow, Cat was able to delegate jobs so that they each had their own little niche in which to work, but yet close enough that Sarah could see how it all went together.

"Bam!" Cat yelled as they finished, which scared Sarah. "Oh, sorry, don't you ever watch Emeril? You know, the guy who cooks on television!"

"No, I like to watch Paula Deen. She is Southern. You should have seen her on Oprah! It was a riot! Eggs and butter all over the place! Oprah was such a good sport about it."

Maria suggested they sit down and have a cup of coffee and rest a spell. "Cat, use the new cups," she suggested.

"Oh, my gosh . . ." Cat yelled.

"What's the matter? Did you break one of my new cups?" Maria hoped not!

"No, but *cups*. We forgot to tell Sarah about the bra and about Betty!" Cat didn't know yet what had happened in the morning hours between Bertha and Sherrie, but when she filled Sarah in on the escapades and her worries about Betty's welfare when Bertha would undoubtedly take up the cause, Sarah offered her brief observations from the lobby.

"All I know is that Bertha was nowhere to be seen when I went through on my way here. I saw a note on the office door that said that Sherrie had gone home with a migraine, and *The Bird Woman* . . . I mean Blanche, was pushing the grocery cart out the door, and I invited her to the potluck. You know, a personal invitation gives a nice touch. I reminded her that since she was the new lady, she didn't have to bring anything this time. I didn't see another soul, so I imagine everyone else was cooking."

"Winnie is probably making her jello," Cat said. "Red or green." Cat and Maria said the last three words in unison and with laughter.

"If she has any sense, she'll be making red for Valentine's Day," Sarah added. "Oh, and by the way, there is no bra on the bulletin board now. I always glance at it. Of course, this morning it was quick look-see, as I was anxious to get in to be with you two, but I would surely have seen a bra!"

"Oh, yes, you would have seen it! It was huge! I can't imagine anyone being that big. Betty had it in here yesterday to show us! They reminded me of the tea cups at the Disneyland ride," Maria said, as she sipped her coffee from the delicate tea cups. "I like dainty, little cups, don't you, Sarah?"

Bras were a touchy subject with Sarah, but she tried to make light of the matter. She unbuttoned her blouse part way. "See, I have my apartment key on a chain right down between my one boob. Ha, Ha. Well, it's not really all that funny; I had breast cancer, in other words."

Maria was ashamed of herself. "That was so insensitive of me, Sarah. I had no idea!"

Sarah waved it off. "At least it's not too obvious that I am . . . well, *challenged,* shall we say, in that area. My gentleman friend has never even noticed it, and he is such a gentleman that he keeps his hands to himself. Oh, did I tell you that he is coming to the potluck? You will get to meet him. I hope it is okay that I invited him; I forgot to write it on the sign-up sheet, but there is always plenty of food. Speaking of food, I'd better get my chicken going. It was frozen solid when I left this morning, but, of course, I can thaw it in the micro. Aren't they wonderful inventions? I use mine all the time, don't you, Maria?"

Maria's long, hard look at Cat said, "Don't you dare say a word!" She'd learn to use it just to keep up with Sarah.

"Yes, I couldn't live without it." Maria nodded in agreement with Sarah. "See you in the Community Room around sixish."

"I'll be there with bells on and with Jess." Sarah finally identified her beau. "Maybe by then you will have figured out your Valentine, or he'll make himself known." Sarah winked and said, "Thanks for the cooking lesson. Ta Ta," and she was out the door.

Maria was exhausted when Sarah left. "What a morning! Are you as tired as I am, Cat? Let's go for a drive and get a mocha before it's time to heat up the cannelloni."

Cat agreed and grabbed their lightweight jackets. The sun was cutting a swath through the trees on the golf course and warming the living room nicely. Cat closed the window that was still open from the cooking session.

"What is that smell?" Maria turned up her nose, as they entered the hallway. "I hope nobody is cooking cabbage or Brussels sprouts for the potluck. It sure is stinking up the place. Do you smell it?"

"Yes, I do smell something, but it's sort of a blended smell of chili and other aromas."

Cat almost gagged, though, as they stood by the bulletin board. "Oh, it's getting stronger and it smells like sewage!" The lobby was quiet, except for Tony who came dashing down the hallway of the west wing with a plunger and plumber's snake.

"Bad news. Winnie's toilet backed up and the sewage is coming up in her bathtub. Sorry to be rude, but I am in a hurry. See you two at the potluck." Tony almost knocked over Otis and Oscar who were coming out of the laundry room with two baskets of clean underwear and towels.

Serves her right, Maria thought, but why did it have to happen today? Tony will have to clear the air with big fans before the potluck.

"What is going on?" Cat knew something was up by her mother's mischievous smile.

"Didn't you hear Tony? He is coming to the potluck."

"So, he must like his daddy's chili." Cat thought it was great for Tony to join his father.

"Or maybe . . . maybe Tony is . . ." Maria let her idea dangle as Cat left her on the bench outside while she went to get the car.

CHAPTER ELEVEN

The Potluck

"A man hath no better thing
Under the sun than to eat,
And to drink and to be merry."
—Ecclesiastes 8:15

Preparations were taking place all over the building while Cat and Maria were out and about. Betty had finally gotten over her night's adventures and was decorating for the potluck. The Community Room had sported a heart motif for a week with cut-outs of hearts on the walls and cupids on the tables. She placed red tablecloths on each table for the special dinner and candles—two on each of the long tables. Some were left over from last Christmas and had more of a holly berry smell than anything else, but what are Valentine's candles supposed to smell like anyway? Any aroma would be better than what was stinkin' up the place as she decorated!

Tony worked quickly and soon had Winnie's bathroom back in good working order.

"What were you trying to flush down there, anyway?" Tony asked.

Winnie hadn't planned on being civil to anyone for the rest of the day, so she snapped back with, "None of your business!"

Millie was indisposed for most of the day. She hadn't even discovered the Valentine on her doorknob. She had gulped down her hot prune juice cocktail in the morning hours and was staying close to home until potluck time. It wouldn't take her long to dump the cheese curls in her prettiest glass bowl, put her dressy, white hearing aids in, and do her face.

And then there were the twins. This was the highlight of the month for them. They had sent away for new sweaters—matching, of course, and had been watching the mail for three weeks in hopes they would show up in time to wear to the potluck. They had arrived the day before, and Oscar and Otis had tried them on immediately and modeled for each other.

The ad had said they were "100% Pure Shetland Wool, Button-Front Cardigans in a rich, deep heather blue reminiscent of the sea, skillfully knit with ribbed cuffs, patch pockets, and a bottom hem." They were the most expensive and luxurious sweaters the twins had ever owned—not at all like the thin, dark blue ones they'd worn for 30 years at the post office.

"These will be our last sweaters," Otis had stated sadly. "We might as well splurge for once in our lives."

Oscar agreed, even though he was tighter with his pennies than Otis. "I'll buy yours if you'll buy mine. That way I will feel better about it, like it's a gift and not just something for myself," rationalizing the price of $69.95 per sweater.

Upstairs on the second floor, Antonio was making his chili, and Tony popped in to taste it several times during the day. "It needs a little more green pepper, Pop," or "Whoa, tone it down. We'll all be having to chew on Tums for dessert."

Others throughout the building were preparing foods, as well, and grooming for the big night. For the couples, it was more than likely the only way they would be celebrating the day for lovers. Some had no way to get to the store to get cards or the money to lavish on a spouse.

Sarah decided to rest in her recliner around two o'clock. Jess was coming at five for a glass of wine before they went down at six for dinner, so she thought she'd sneak in a bit of shut-eye and still have time to cook the chicken, but when she woke up at four p.m., she knew she was doomed.

In panic, she dialed Jess's number. "You'd never guess what happened to me," she sheepishly told him. "I had a . . . a lengthy appointment this afternoon, and now it is too late to cook for the potluck. Do you suppose you could pick up some KFC on your way here? You'd better get a lot—like twelve pieces . . . . No, no, not a whole dinner, just a bucket of chicken. And you know I like the breasts. I don't want a rib, a neck, or an artery!"

Maria and Cat drove over to Albertson's, so Cat could pick up a few personal items and *The Oregonian*, the big newspaper from the Portland area, and who should they run into but Betty and Gayle. They were coming out of the bakery department with a beautifully decorated, large sheet cake—with red roses on pink frosting for Valentine's Day.

When Betty saw them, her first reaction was, "No matter what I do, I get caught."

She went on to explain that Gayle and she were bringing this surprise to the potluck, and she had hoped nobody would know who supplied it. "Our treat. We're both cutting back on our smoking, so we had a little extra money this month and could splurge, but now, don't tell."

"We won't tell. What a nice gesture!" Maria was quick to praise them. "But, good luck sneaking it in through the lobby. The spies will be out!"

Gayle assured them that the plan was to go in the back door that opened into the Community Room and set it on the dessert table early before others showed up. "We know it's hard to keep anything a secret, but we'll try. We can always say we were picking it up for someone else, and then that would really stir up the soup kettle with wonder."

They all paid for their items and went out the door together. Maria and Cat were back in time to heat up the cannelloni and to get dressed for the potluck. They had no idea what to wear. Cat doubted if anyone gussied up much, but Maria reminded her that, after all, it was Valentine's Day, so at the very least, they should both wear red.

"Oh yes, to match Winnie's red jello." Cat threw in, "unless she brings green, and then we won't be color-coordinated!"

"She has no idea how much humor we've gotten out of her potluck offering on the sign-up sheet, has she?" Maria laughed, as she pulled on her pair of good, black slacks.

"Probably not, but we have to find something to laugh about. I had no idea retirement homes were like this. I just wonder if they all are." Cat shook her head and grimaced, as she helped her mom button up a long-sleeved red blouse.

"I don't know, but there are a lot of us old, mixed nuts running around, and just wait until all you baby-boomers get old enough to need a place to hang your hat. I probably won't live to see that, but it will be interesting."

Cat's remark in reply competed with the oven bell ringing, "Yeah, I'll say *hello* to a fellow cashew now and then for you, Mom, my favorite nut!"

*　　*　　*

And so the long-awaited potluck began. There was no seating order, but it was noticeable that some seating arrangements had either been planned in advance or else a certain person just happened to show up at the opportune time to conveniently find a place next to someone with whom he or she really wanted to dine. Several had signed up Saturday afternoon, so their contributions for the dinner were a surprise.

Oscar and Otis arrived early. They hadn't read the revised sign-up sheet, and Oscar brought a small cake, which paled in comparison to the large cake and looked lost on the big dessert table, but Betty politely thanked Oscar for it. The twins, who often ate silently and alone, sat with Millie, as did Antonio. That was undoubtedly the most glaring difference from previous dinners, and eyes darted to and fro, trying not to stare, but not wanting to miss a moment of this new development. The twins were actually socializing!

Tony sat with Maria and Cat, which they thought was unusual, since he had come with his dad, but they figured Tony could see that Dad didn't need his son around tonight. "I was sure your sweetie would want to sit with you," Cat whispered to Maria.

"Be quiet! See, I told you he wasn't my sweetie!" Maria smugly said.

Sarah arrived with Jess, who carried in her platter of fried chicken nicely arranged with sprigs of parsley interspersed. They sat with several other couples.

Essie brought her green salad, but Winnie and her jello salad did not show up. This was the first potluck Winnie had ever missed. Some were glad to be free of her roving eyes, but Essie missed her and wondered where she could possibly be. "You know, once I took a big spoonful of the topping on her jello and put it in mouth all at once. I thought it was Cool Whip, but guess what? It was Miracle Whip!" Essie said to Maria, who was seated next to her.

"That *would* be a surprise," Maria looked wisely at Cat, but Cat was deep into conversation with Tony.

The last two to arrive were Bertha with a small, garden salad, and Blanche with nothing. Blanche had been out most of the afternoon with the grocery cart, retrieving the last of her possessions from the storage unit. She was late and wind-blown and had returned to her nest to wash her hands and don a clean pair of jeans. She parked the grocery cart just outside the door of the Community Room, since there was no way she could bring it in and put it in the store room with the potluck in full swing. Bertha deposited her salad near Essie's and wheeled over and parked by the dessert table where she had a view of the entire room. No one offered her a spot at their table, so she finally wangled her wheelchair to the end of a table where she barely knew anyone. She didn't care! She would rather eat alone than have to converse with these ingrates. They didn't appreciate all she tried to do for them anyway.

Paul Clairmont, a retired pastor and a widower down past Bertha's apartment, offered the blessing, and then Betty invited everyone to "dig in, folks."

The line moved quickly, everyone seemed to enjoy the selections of dishes, and the food disappeared in a hurry. The cannelloni received rave reviews. Even Bertha liked it.

"All that work, and now it's gone. Just like on Thanksgiving. We used to cook for hours when the family was home, and they ate so fast to get back in the family room to watch football. At least here they are staying and visiting over cake and coffee," Maria observed and tried to tell Cat, but she had tuned her out. Tony had her full attention.

If awards had been given out for the best dressed couple, they surely would have gone to Oscar and Otis for their new sweaters. Their hair looked clean, and even if some dandruff had fallen, it would have been inconspicuous and blended in better than on that dark blue of their common, ordinary sweaters. They shyly accepted all the compliments and Oscar, especially, smiled more than he had in years. Millie's smile was tugging on his heart strings, and for someone who had rarely dated and never married, that was an odd sensation to be happening so late in life for Oscar. In fact, he thought he could be having a heart attack!

Essie had come over to eat dessert with Bertha. "Look at those two old coots. Isn't that ridiculous at their ages?" Bertha pointed at Oscar and Millie, who were really doing nothing to cause such a stir. Antonio was vying for Millie's attention, as well.

"This is a terrible thing to say, but my sister always said," Essie chimed in, "'Men are hot-blooded until the day they die, and even then I wonder . . .'"

Betty was busy serving cake, and Gayle was pouring coffee. They both hoped that someone would help clean up. Even though each person who had brought a covered dish or salad would take their containers home, there were always a few dishes to do, tables to wipe off, and the floor to vacuum. Tony had promised to stay and put the tables and chairs back in their usual arrangement, but Betty was beginning to wonder if he'd even remember. He had not talked to anyone but Cat all evening.

"I'm afraid he's smitten, Gayle," Betty whispered to her helper, who nodded in agreement.

All too soon the Valentine's potluck was over, and the residents and guests started trickling out the door. Maria was receiving compliments on her cannelloni, and one lady from the third floor asked for the recipe. "It was the best dish here," she told Maria, who beamed like the summer sun. "I bet you have lots of good recipes and will bring something good every time."

"That is, . . . if I come," Maria said, as she thanked the lady.

Cat finally noticed that the whole affair was over when her mother struggled to push her chair back to leave. "Oh, are you leaving? Well, um . . . . I, um . . . told Tony I'd help him clean up, so I'll be down in a little while, OK?"

Maria wanted to ask if she had a choice or a say in the matter, but really, when she stopped and thought about it, yes, it was okay. After all, Cat *was* fifty-six years old!

Sarah was holding on to Jess's arm for support, no doubt, and as they left at the same time as Maria, Sarah whispered in her ear, "I see that everyone liked your cannelloni, but no one asked for my chicken recipe. I'm certainly not jealous, but I am just a little bit miffed."

Maria didn't have the heart to tell her that it so obviously looked and tasted like the Colonel's that everyone knew she hadn't outdone herself over a hot stove.

"It was delicious, Sarah. I hope you'll bring it again next time. I'd eat it again, well, that is . . . if I come." Maria had only come this time because of Cat, and now she was going home alone!

Bertha maintained her perch at the end of the table, so she could inspect the clean up.

Cat knew *she* didn't want to ask her to move, and Tony tried to work around her, but when the cord of the vacuum got caught in the wheel of her chair, someone had to speak up. Gayle, bless her heart, came to the rescue. "Oh, Bertha, I wonder if you'd come here for a minute and hold this Saran Wrap at one end, so I can cover the cake. In fact, I'll get a paper plate, and you can take some of it home for a late night snack." Gayle undid the vacuum cord and turned Bertha's wheelchair in the direction of the dessert table. She and Bertha had never seen eye to eye, but Gayle was an expert in diplomacy and had a forgiving heart.

"Gayle, if I've told you once, I've told you a dozen times that I am diabetic. I couldn't eat that cake with all that gooey frosting. Who brought it, anyway?"

Gayle had noticed that Bertha had a small piece of Oscar's chocolate cake, but apparently that didn't count. Gayle handled it well, saying, "Oh yes, I am so sorry; I totally forgot, Bertha. Here, grab this end and we'll cover the cake. I suppose we could put it out in the morning for the Koffee Klatch. What do you think?"

"Well, if you want my opinion, and obviously you do or you wouldn't have asked, I think it is a good idea to get rid of it as soon as possible. It could attract mice, you know."

Bertha was springing back to form. "Who did you say brought it?"

Gayle ignored Bertha's question both times, but she assured her that she would refrigerate it over night, so it would be safe. Betty completely ignored Bertha, and if Bertha made any smart remarks to her, she would throw her dishrag in the sink and leave. Bertha could finish the dishes and be the director!

Meanwhile, Maria made it home unescorted. She found it hard to believe that her highly intelligent daughter had picked up with the maintenance man, but she had learned long ago to keep quiet about Cat's affairs. "I just hope she comes home early tonight; she will soon be gone, and I will be so all alone," Maria said aloud, as she put the casserole dish in the sink to be washed at a later date.

The potluck was over at 7:30 and Cat didn't return until almost 10:00. She tiptoed in, hoping her mother would be asleep, but Maria had fought off the sandman's attempts, and was seated in her usual spot at the far end of the couch.

Maria stifled a yawn. "So, you're finally here. That must have been one dirty Community Room! But, oh well, sit down here by me; I have so much to tell you."

"Well, so do I, but you go first." Cat wasn't too eager to tell her mother of the plans she had made for Saturday night, while she and Tony were out looking at his Ford truck and telling Antonio "good night" in his apartment.

"OK. Here goes. First of all, look at the box of candy on the coffee table. That was propped up against my door when I got home from the potluck. So, what do you think about that?" She had no idea who the sneaky Cupid could be.

"Wow, you do have a sweetie, but who? None of the eligible bachelors paid any attention to you at the potluck. Oh, was there a card?" Cat thought that might solve it.

"Yes, right here. I had to get the magnifying glass out to read it because the print was so small. I think it says 'Grow old along with me! The best is yet to be, The last of life, for which the first was made—Our times are in his hand.'"

Cat nodded and smiled. "By Robert Browning. I have always loved that little verse. You must have a very romantic sweetie, Mom!"

"Yes, but who is he?" Once again, there was no signature. Maria did not like secrets or the unknown, and so by process of elimination, she and Cat ran down the list of the men that they knew of up and down the hallways. They really had only met Antonio and Tony, and they ruled them both out, although Tony had admitted that he had left the other candies and the card for Cat. Otis, Oscar, and Antonio all seemed enthralled with Millie, so that apparently left them out. "I hope this all ends now that Valentine's Day is over; it is just ridiculous, especially since I just moved in here. Nobody really knows me!"

They finally gave up and went on to Maria's other bit of news.

"There was a message from Jillian on my machine when I walked in tonight. She invited us over for dinner tomorrow night. Michael will cook, as usual. It's too late to call her back now, but I'll tell her "yes" first thing in the morning. Okay?"

Cat hemmed and hawed and stalled with her answer. "Well, um, maybe could we go on Sunday? I was going to leave Sunday, but could wait until the next day. I'm um . . . a . . . sort of busy tomorrow night."

Maria was more shocked that Cat had planned to leave Sunday than she was about her busy Saturday night schedule. She had tried to shove it back into the recesses of her mind, as she had done with so many things her whole life, but here it was, about to happen.

"No, they're busy Sunday. Michael has a golf tournament in the morning, and then they are going to *her* mother's for dinner later on, so it's tomorrow night or nothing. What is so pressing with you, anyway, that you can't go to your brother's?" Maria was upset and wide awake.

Cat blurted it out and got it over with. "Tony and I are going out to dinner. There is a little Italian restaurant near Albertson's. He says their food is 'authentically Italian'. Isn't that almost poetic? Don't you just love it?"

"Authentic, poetic, pathetic—whatever. Okay, I'll just have to tell Jillian we'll have to do it next time you come to town. Oh, I just thought of something. Now that you have a sweetie, you'll probably be coming quite often, and that will be nice. I just hope you'll have some time to spend with your poor old mama."

Cat was quick to set her mother straight. "Mom, come on. I just met him, and it's Valentine's Day. It doesn't mean a thing. He just wanted to celebrate the day today, and one little dinner tomorrow doesn't mean anything. After all, we have to eat!"

Maria was yawning again and thought Cat's logic for the next night's date was so far out that it was illogical. "Oh, well, what the heck! Let's go to bed.

We wouldn't want you to be up too late and have bags under your eyes, now would we? Tony wouldn't like that!"

Maria was about to say "good night" when she remembered the Koffee Klatch in the morning. "One more thing, Cat. Are we going to the Koffee Klatch? If so, I have nothing to take, and oh, we need to get your laundry done tomorrow, too. I won't send you home dirty!"

"I can run and get some donuts in the morning, if we decide to go. Don't worry about it, Mom." She knew Maria would wake up all night and stew about it. "On second thought, maybe I should get some fruit instead. Gayle put the cake in the refrigerator for the morning's get-together."

Maria was shocked. "Cake for breakfast? What is this place coming to?"

CHAPTER TWELVE

Winnie Disappears

"Unique Walking Stick. Rubber-tipped
Walking companion complete with
Corded glass bottle for your favorite liquid.
Designed in three sections for easy packing."

With the potluck behind them, many of the thirty-nine residents (Bertha had counted), were either too exhausted or still feeling too full to gather again Saturday morning for the Koffee Klatch. Of course, there were only a handful of regulars on any given Saturday, so it was not unusual for a small turn-out on the "morning after the night before."

Betty and Gayle were always there early to make the coffee—one pot of decaf and one of regular coffee. They also put out small plates and napkins and greeted the arrivals.

The phone had been busy at Maria's. She called Jillian as soon as she thought they would be up, but she was too late; they had already gone to the boys' soccer game. Her message was short and to the point. "Cat has already made other plans for us Saturday night, so unless you can work in a visit on Sunday somehow, she will have to see you all next time. Bye." She didn't mean to be terse or sound upset: she just didn't want to give an explanation.

She had just put the phone down when Sarah called to tell her that she would not be going to the Koffee Klatch. "I am in a bad way this morning. In fact, I'm not even dressed. I ate too much and ate all the wrong things, so my stomach is all torn up today. Oh, now, don't get the wrong idea and think it was your cannelloni. I made the mistake of eating that chili and Bertha's salad. I should know better. It's just too much roughage! Oh, but how are you, Maria? Are you going down the hall for a little bit of breakfast and gossip?"

"Yes, we are going as soon as Cat gets back. I sent her to the store to get some fruit. I wanted to take some cinnamon rolls from the bakery down the street, but changed my tune on that when Cat said that Gayle was putting out the left-over cake. Can you imagine? Cake for breakfast?" Maria was still shocked at the thought of it and how it had changed her plans. She had never liked change, and now in her *golden years* it was even more difficult to adapt. She liked her word—*stick-to-it-iv-ness*. Most didn't have it in today's world.

Sarah wondered what the difference was between cinnamon rolls that usually were covered with sweet frosting or a cake, but all she said was, "Oh, yes, all that sugar. That's why I try to walk around the building as soon as the Klatch is over, but I will be skipping that today, too. Well, I must go and take some Imodium, Maria, so you and Cat have fun. Don't do anything I wouldn't do! Ta, Ta."

Thank goodness she didn't ask any questions about receiving Valentines, Maria thought, as she waited for Cat. She didn't want to listen to any gossip this morning either.

Bertha, Essie, Betty, Gayle, and Blanche were the only ones seated around a table when Maria and Cat entered the Community Room with a bowl of seedless grapes and some apple quarters on a small tray. Bertha had decided to tolerate Betty temporarily.

"Have a seat, girls. Oh, red and green grapes to make up for Winnie's lack of jello last night?" Betty observed with laughter.

"No, I didn't plan it that way," Maria said, never giving the color scheme a thought.

"By the way, where is Winnie? She wasn't here last night, and, of course, this is my first Saturday morning, so I don't know if she comes to this or not."

Bertha had an answer, although it was incomplete, for a change. "Oh, she's gone again. I was worried about her, and when she didn't answer her phone last night, I went down to her place this morning. She has given me a spare key, so I knocked and then went in." She stopped abruptly and they all thought that was the unfinished end to her story. She was thinking, wondering how much to tell their hungry ears.

"Well . . . go on. Tell us more." Blanche twittered, as she perched on the edge of her chair. The little bird woman was like a baby wren waiting while the mother bird dangled a worm in front of her. It was all news to her, since she was the current *new lady*.

"Her place was all cleaned up. Sometimes it's a mess with, well . . . um . . . bottles around. I guess I don't have to tell you that she has a drinking problem. But today it was spotless, and the awful stench from yesterday's plumbing problem was totally gone, as well. In fact, the strong smell of Clorox took my breath away!"

Cat decided to jump into the story. "Oh yes, Tony said it was awful to go into that apartment. She wouldn't tell him what she had tried to flush down her toilet, and it was out of sight when he got there. He said that it must have been something big! But that doesn't answer the burning question of where she went." Cat was interested, too. She was always looking for fodder for her next novel. She should have brought her notebook.

Bertha continued, "She stomps off with her cane, but never tells anyone where she is going and when she gets back, she is real secretive. She doesn't even tell me where she is going, even though she says I am her only friend here. I can't believe she doesn't tell me."

Bertha's usually stoic face registered a hurt expression. "And she goes for two weeks at a time."

Just then Millie entered the scene. "Have I missed Act I?" she asked, in her affected stage voice. Without fail, she arrived late, and the regulars knew by now it was for effect.

She swooped over to Cat and patted her on the head. "You are up early, dahling. How was your date last night? I saw you out front with Tony. Isn't he marvelous and so handsome? He should be on the silver screen. You're so lucky to have found each other!"

Cat was speechless, so she just smiled and hoped someone would change the subject.

"We were just talking about Winnie. She has disappeared again. Have you seen her, Millie?" Betty came to her rescue.

"What did she say?" Millie whispered to Maria, as she sat down next to her. "I took out my hearing aids last night, and now I can't find them."

"So what else is new! You say that every Saturday, Millie. Why don't you put them in one place where you'll always know where they are?" Bertha's disgust with Millie was wearing her down all ready, and she was ready to wheel away to her apartment. "My care-giver is coming later on, and I have to get things in order. I'm so glad I have a good excuse to leave all of you to try to figure out where Winnie went," she added sarcastically.

Gayle insisted she take some cake home for the care-giver. Bertha wanted two pieces, and they all knew her care-giver would be lucky to get any. Bertha cheated and played games with her diabetes and thought no one was the wiser.

Just as they were starting to gossip about Oscar and Otis, Maria put her left hand up to her puffy left earlobe, and then she touched her right one with her other hand. "Oh, my gosh! I'm naked. I have to go home right now! Come on, Cat."

Cat quelled the questioning looks by saying, "Yes, girls, she forgot her earrings, and she never leaves home without them!"

CHAPTER THIRTEEN

Cat's Last Day

"Whenever I prepare for a journey
I prepare as though for death.
Should I never return, all is in order.
This is what life has taught me."
—Katherine Mansfield

The dirty wash . . . Cat had never figured out why her mother called it that. Of course it was dirty. No one would wash clean clothes, but when Maria told Cat to gather up the *dirty wash*, she didn't question her. With it all in two laundry baskets, mother and daughter struggled out the apartment door and down the hallway shortly after coming back from the Koffee Klatch. The disturbance in the library caught them by surprise.

Bertha was all over Sarah for forgetting to pick up Friday night's newspaper. Maria was surprised to see that Sarah was out and about since she'd *been in a bad way* earlier, and she thought Bertha would be busy with her care-giver.

They didn't know what all had ensued, but they heard Bertha's voice as she spotted them and left the library. "Never fear, Sarah. I will not wait for the next Association meeting to bring your laxness out in the open. First thing Monday morning, you know where I'll be!"

Sarah plopped down hard on a wooden chair by the long table where the papers and magazines waited to be picked up and read. "Oh, Maria and Cat, I've never been happier to see anyone in my whole life! Did you hear that? It's no wonder I am in a bad way all the time. She makes me so nervous! I remembered the paper this morning, but I had to wait for my Imodium to kick in before I ventured out." Sarah rubbed her forehead, and she hoped she wasn't getting a headache to accompany her other problems.

"She is a stern taskmaster; I can see that. If she could get out of the wheelchair, she could be in law enforcement." Maria had set her laundry basket down just inside the door, and she patted Sarah on the shoulder. "Come on down and visit with us while we do the dirty laundry. We'll put the clothes in and then sit in the lobby and visit and hope no one disturbs us. Come on," she encouraged Sarah again.

"I guess I could. There is a bathroom right by the laundry room . . . just in case. Jess said he would call today, but I don't know when. Oh well, he can call back." Sarah chatted away all the way through the lobby and into the laundry room, and she continued on while Maria and Cat sorted the clothes and filled two machines, even though she didn't like to talk. The other two washers were apparently finished with their wash cycles, but obviously in use. Maria hadn't learned yet that Saturday was a busy wash day nor did she know how lucky she was to find two machines available.

"Put the quarters in, Cat, and we'll go set a spell." Cat filled two slots and pushed the wash cycle buttons to breathe life into two machines.

The two comfortable upholstered chairs in the lobby were on each side of a lamp table, so Cat was left standing when Maria and Sarah were seated, and it made it hard for all three to visit. But, Cat, still having an agile body, plopped down on the floor in front of them, much to her mother's consternation. As others stopped by to visit, they stood, and soon the circle was full. Sarah introduced Maria and Cat to a couple ladies from up on her floor, and the time passed quickly.

Cat excused herself and went to check on the laundry. How odd, she thought, as she put up the lid on one of the machines. The clothes were as dry as an old lady's skin and hadn't moved. The other machine had finished the cycles, and the clothes were ready to be transferred to a dryer.

As Cat was contemplating what to do, a lady she had never seen before entered the room and threw up the lid of the machine next to Maria's and said in a whiney voice, "I don't know what is wrong with this machine; it never gets done! I left here an hour or so ago, and look, it is just now on the spin cycle."

Cat agreed with her that the machines were not in good working order and told her about how one of her washers hadn't even started yet.

The whiney lady wandered off to the bathroom and said she'd be right back, and Cat decided to put more quarters in and see what would happen.

The machines were close together—almost touching each other—and as Cat began to place the quarters in the slots, she realized that the first time she had put them in the whiney lady's machine by mistake!

She could blame it on Sarah and her babbling on and ruining her concentration, but worse yet, she was afraid she was becoming a *mixed nut*, just by association. Surely it takes more than one week, she mused, as she sheepishly made her way out to the group of ladies.

Maria wanted a detailed account of how the laundry was progressing, but Cat just said it was going very well. There was no way she was going to tell these women what she had done. Later, she would tell her mother who would predictably be upset at first, but soon when she would describe the whiney lady's disbelief, Maria would think it was hilarious.

And as they were putting the clean laundry away, that is just what happened. "I can see you would fit right in here, Cat. Why don't you stay longer?" Maria strongly suggested.

Cat predicted that, as well. Her mother would be begging her to extend her visit or even move in, but they had to make the break sometime, and Cat was going to stick to leaving on Sunday, no matter what anyone said or did.

They went out for one final mocha in the early afternoon and for a short drive around the city. It was unusually warm for the middle of February, and Cat wanted to pop the top on the convertible and let the light breeze ruffle through her short, curly hair, but Maria had a fit. "I just got my hair done, Cat. Lord knows when I'll get back in there for a perm, and besides, all that wind is not good for your hair. It just dries it up, and you want to look nice for your big date tonight, don't you?"

Cat could see by the look on her mother's face and by the tone of her voice that depression was already trying to worm its way into her being. She knew her mother wanted her to stay home with her for a quiet meal and conversation, but she had promised to see Tony just this one time.

In desperation she blurted out, "Oh, Mom, I just had a brilliant idea. Why don't you and Antonio join us for dinner? We can double-date! Wouldn't that be fun?!"

Maria had just taken a sip of her iced mocha, and when she snorted, it came out her nose. "Now look what you've done; I could have choked to death. Cat, why don't you think before you talk like that? And quit playing matchmaker! I can handle my own affairs!"

Cat knew she had said the wrong thing, so she let the word *affairs* die on her mother's lips. Her creative spirit could have taken the ball and run in for a touchdown with that one word, but instead, as she rounded the corner and turned into the parking lot at Pear Blossom, she saw the square, box-shaped vehicle and flashing lights that unmistakably was an ambulance parked in the driveway right in front of the entrance. Those vehicles never stood for anything happy or good going on, and she knew that her mother would be panic-stricken to think that one of her neighbors was being hauled away.

Cat pulled in behind it, but kept at a safe distance. For once she was glad that her mother's eyesight was far from 20/20, and she couldn't see the victim on the gurney. Cat didn't know who it was, but she assured her mother that it was probably no one they knew and was probably just a precautionary measure—nothing really very serious. Oh boy, this is all she needs to send her into a fearful depression and with me leaving tomorrow, Cat thought as the ambulance pulled away and her mother got out to wait on the bench while Cat parked the car down the row in the visitor's section.

The lobby was as deserted as if it were the middle of the night, which made Cat and Maria extremely happy. Neither one really wanted to hear details or identity of the person that was just taken away, although Maria prayed it was no one she had met. Somehow that made it just a bit easier if she hadn't made the person's acquaintance.

"Maybe I should stay home with you tonight, Mom, and not go out with Tony," Cat said, as she could sense her mother's anxiety and the sadness that was drowning in the lines of her cheeks. At least there were no tears just yet.

"I should say not! You go and have some fun. I'll just whoop it up with Lawrence Welk, and Daniel O' Donnell has a Valentine's show, and you know how I love him."

"Yes, we know that *he* is your sweetie, for sure!" Cat just loved to throw that word around.

Both ladies jumped at the knock on the door, even though Tony was expected at any moment. Cat was still busy preparing for the big date, so Maria answered the door.

Expecting to see a tall man maybe holding a bouquet of flowers, Maria looked up, but no, it was short, little Betty wondering if Maria and Cat would like to play cards in the Community Room after dinner.

"Oh gosh, I just don't know, Betty. Cat is going out tonight, and I can't see too well to play games, and my shows are on and . . ."

Cat had heard all of this from the bedroom. "Yes, she would love to play cards, Betty. What time should she be there?" Cat was breathing many sighs of relief and could have hugged Betty to death for coming to her rescue.

As it turned out, mother and daughter both had a great time with their evening's adventures. Cat and Tony enjoyed their Italian dinner and whatever else they did. Maria didn't pry or ask as many questions about Cat's evening as Cat did about her mother's card games. Cat and Tony agreed to continue their friendship long-distance with e-mails and phone calls, but Cat brushed it off to her mother like it was no big deal.

Maria was reluctant to show enthusiasm because she never felt like she was having a really good time, and tonight of all nights with Cat leaving tomorrow, she should show more sadness, but she couldn't help but tell Cat about her evening. "That Betty is a corker. We played UNO, and every time she had to draw 4 cards or got skipped, she'd yell, 'May the bird of paradise fly up your nose.' Plus, Betty made daiquiris, and I had two!"

"Well, no wonder you had a good time. No need to worry about you. I go out for an innocent, little dinner and you get snockered!" Cat jabbed and poked to get her mother all riled up.

Maria took umbrage with that word *snockered*. "I shpose you're goin' to tell me you didn't have wine with your dinner." She tried to slur her words and staggered over to the couch. She hiccupped for added effect.

"Oh, Mom, you are so funny! You can't even pretend to be a good drunk!"

"That's because I've never had much practice. Lord knows, if I would have tried to keep up with your father and all his cocktails, I'd have been an annual visitor at the Betty Ford Clinic." Maria grimaced with disdain at the thought of her late-husband's bad habit.

"Maybe that's where Winnie goes now and then," Cat pondered aloud, wanting to dismiss any derogatory conversation about her father, who had been her hero, in spite of his sinful ways. He had left this earth 12 years ago, and Cat still missed him with a passion.

"No, I don't think so. The girls were saying she says things like 'I had an appointment with destiny,' or 'My investments were going south,' or the weirdest one of all—'I was following the magnetic pull,' so see, who knows what she is doing. We all wondered at UNO tonight if she even knows herself what she is doing."

"Yeah, she's a tough nut to crack, all right!" Cat tried to sum her all up and put her in the can with the other mixed nuts. She was tired and ready for bed. Yes, she and Tony had shared a bottle of wine with their dinner, and sleep was begging for admittance.

Maria, on the other hand, although sleepy, did not want the day or the week or Cat's visit to end, but morning knocked once again in a few short hours and banged her way into their dream-filled worlds to taste reality. Maria fought hard to keep her eyelids closed to block out the vision of the day that Cat was leaving, but as hard as she tried, the pull of the morning sunlight tugged them open. She could smell coffee and heard Cat rumbling around in the living room—both a delight to her senses. Funny how a person could get so used to the comforting smells and sounds in such a short time, especially when she had lived alone for so many years. She loved how Cat somehow had a way about her that calmed Maria's anxieties, and she knew what to say and do, even if she didn't know how to put quarters in a washing machine. Her own daughter was two quarters short of a full load! Maria chuckled at that story once again as she struggled from the bed sheets and planted her feet on the beige carpet of her bedroom.

"What is so funny?" Cat threw open the door and glanced in at the old woman in her nightgown sitting on the edge of her bed. She looked tousled and forlorn, and Cat wondered if she had lost her senses in the middle of the night. She had expected trouble and tears, not giggles from her mother.

Maria pointed a crooked, bony finger at Cat. "Oh, I just woke up thinking about you washing clothes yesterday, and that poor old woman thinking her machine was broken. Cat, you just need to learn how to get your ducks in a row."

Cat looked at her mother in consternation.

"Oh, yes, I know, I used a cliche—ducks in a row—and I know how you writers hate clichés, but we old people have used them all our lives, and sometimes they just say the right thing so perfectly." Maria felt like babbling on like Sarah; maybe time would stop and Cat would stay if she was held under the sway of words. "Foolishness!" Maria said loudly.

Cat didn't know what was going on with her mother. "What is foolishness?"

"Oh, just me, thinking that maybe I could talk you into staying longer. So, just get ready and go and get it over with." Maria's light mood had vanished, not to be seen again that day.

"The good news is, Mom, that I'll be back in April. Tony wants me to come down for the Pear Blossom Festival." Cat smiled as she told her mother, who had shuffled to her spot in the corner of the couch near the window.

Oh, so it's what Tony wants now, Maria thought, not when I might need her. She gazed out at the golf course, not seeing much of anything. She took a sip of coffee and banged the cup down on the coffee table much too loudly.

"What's wrong?" Cat wondered aloud. She already knew the answer, but heard a different one that didn't ring true.

"Oh, I'll be so busy by then with everything that goes on here. I probably won't have time to visit much. My social calendar will be full, but, of course, you can stay here, and we'll run into each other now and then." Maria choked out the last few words and covered her face. The veins of her hand looked like a map of the Los Angeles freeway, and her throat was just as congested as those highways.

Cat rushed to her side. "I know it's hard, Mom, and I know you are trying. Now, be the trooper, the strong one in the family that you've always been." She pulled her mother's hands away from her face and took Maria's cheeks in her own hands. "I can come whenever you need me, okay? And if I know my sisters, surely Gabby and Gina will want to come and see where their mom is living now, plus Michael and Jillian are just across town, and maybe even Laura will be able to come some day."

Maria looked into Cat's eyes that were ablaze with sincerity and with faith that Maria could handle it all in due time. Maria read the trust that Cat would keep her word, and that her other grown children would indeed come to see her. Cat's hopes were Maria's lifeline.

"Gotta go now, Mom. I'll call you when I get home and call you every day," Cat hollered over her shoulder as she rolled her suitcases out the door and into the hallway.

She felt the pull of emotion, too and ran back to kiss her mother good-bye.

Just as she was entering the lobby with her luggage, Sarah disembarked from the elevator.

"What a godsend you are, Sarah!" Cat was the one who gushed this time. "Are you going out today?" she added, hoping that Sarah could help her calm her fears about her mother.

"Why, yes, I am. I'm waiting for Jess to pick me up for church, and then we are going to the Bountiful Buffet. I shouldn't go and eat all that food. You know, because of my hiatal hernia and reflux, so I'll just have to be careful. Oh, why did you ask?"

Cat jumped in while she could. "Do you think on your way home from the buffet that you could possibly stop somewhere and get my mother an iced mocha? They really perk her up, and she'll need a boost today. She suffers from depression, you know. She's had problems off and on with it for years."

Sarah's face was stricken with concern. "Oh, I'm so sorry; I had no idea. But, yes, Cat, you can count on me to be her friend, and of course, we will get her that mocha."

Cat grabbed Sarah's hand and was pressing a ten-dollar bill into it. "Here is some money, and you'd better get her a double shot and get yourself a drink, too."

"Shot? What do you mean by shot?" Sarah was not up on all the java terminology. "You see, Cat, I don't drink those milky drinks. You know, with my lactose intolerance problem."

Is there nothing that you don't have physically wrong with you? Cat wondered to herself.

"Shot means how much coffee they put in it. Mom needs a jolt of caffeine, so two shots today, and you could drink them if you ordered soy milk. The secret is in the soy."

Sarah put her arm around Cat as they walked to the door. "Now, don't worry, Cat. I will save the extra money and get her another one someday when I'm out, and I'll check on her and cheer her up. I know what it's like to be depressed. After my husband died, I was so . . . Oh, there's Jess! Have a safe trip, Cat, and come back soon. I'll get the latte." She waved, as she got in Jess's car.

"No, an iced mocha," Cat yelled, but doubted if Sarah heard her.

*   *   *

Maria could already feel herself swimming into the abyss of depression. Cat had been her anchor that kept the ship afloat, but now when Cat shut the door and left her there alone, the fears of drowning into hopelessness that she'd experienced so many times before washed over her in waves. She closed her eyes and thought of the sad times in her life—how happiness and sadness shifted like the sand that she liked to walk on at the coast. She thought of the baby who had died at birth, the car accident when she was in her 30's that left her with arthritis from so many broken bones, her bittersweet marriage to Grayson and then his untimely death with a sudden heart attack, the loss of her sister to cancer, and on and on and on. Even the most minute events with just a tinge of sadness brought her emotions welling up and spilling over.

Finally, she dozed and her dreams were mixed up and crazy—of people she had never seen before and of places where she'd never been and didn't recognize. She heard knocking but ignored it. She heard ringing—a shrill, jangling ring—but let that go, too, and when she finally woke up, she wasn't sure what was a dream or reality. Her eyes darted around the room, and the emptiness brought her back to the real world.

She struggled to her feet and shuffled to the kitchen to squint at the clock. It was almost noon and here she was, still in her nightgown and no breakfast or lunch. She wasn't hungry, but opened the plastic bread sack that was resting on the counter. She smeared some peanut butter on the crust and went back to her cozy, old familiar corner of the couch. She pulled the afghan up to her chin and snuggled into the corner again. She wanted to hibernate like a bear and not wake up until April. She choked down the bread and then dozed off again, and she was dreaming that she and Cat were on a cruise ship. They were having a great time, but then she lost sight of her daughter. She caught up with her just in time to see Cat falling into the ocean, and she never saw her again.

Maria awoke with a start. Someone was banging on her door. "Is that you, Cat?" She was so confused. Cat was gone, but where? Back on the ship?

The banging continued, and she heard a voice, "Maria, are you there? Maria, answer the door!"

"Who is it?" Maria finally swept away the confusion and stumbled to the door.

"It's Sarah. I have a surprise for you, Maria."

Maria reluctantly opened the door. "Oh, Sarah, I'm not dressed yet," but when she saw the drink, she perked up instantly. "Is that for me? Well, come on in. I'll throw on a bathrobe. I must look a sight. Have a seat," she added, as she pointed to the couch and hurried into the bedroom. Sarah had gotten it right; it was an iced mocha, two shots, and even had whipping cream on the top.

"Where is yours?" Maria asked, as she marched back into the living room with her light blue bathroom tied firmly around her waist. She couldn't wait to have a sip of the mocha.

"Oh, I've never had one. With all my health problems, I just don't think they would agree with me—all that chocolate and milk and caffeine. I'm already in a bad way, you know! In fact, Jess and I just got back from the buffet, and I ate all the wrong things. I told my doctor just the other day that they can split the atom and send a man to the moon, but they can't cure irritable bowel syndrome. He agreed with me and added that they can't cure the common cold either! So, I'd better get home before something happens. You look so comfy, Maria, in your nightgown; I think I'll just get my jammies on and take it easy the rest of the day." Sarah rubbed her abdomen in distress.

Maria had no intention of getting dressed, but pretended to have plans. "I need to get a bath and get some clothes on. I think my son will be calling." The hint for Sarah to take her departure fell on deaf ears.

"Oh yes, I heard you have a son—a dentist. Is that right?" As Maria nodded, Sarah continued. "That reminds me; I must call my dentist. I have one tooth that is really bothering me. You see, I have all my own teeth. Isn't that remarkable for someone my age?" She'd forgotten that she was going home, as she launched into her dental health.

Maria was glad she'd at least put her teeth in that morning before Cat left, and she hoped Sarah wouldn't ask about her dentures.

Twenty minutes later when the phone rang, Sarah and Maria both jumped. Sarah was deep into describing how she had come to know Jess, but when Maria answered the phone and said, "Oh, hello Cat," Sarah recognized her cue to leave.

Sarah whispered into the phone, as she gave Maria's shoulder a good-bye squeeze. "Mission accomplished!"

CHAPTER FOURTEEN

The Senior Project

"If you take things apart,
You find out what they are made of."
—anon

"She doesn't even like herself." Those words that Sarah had spoken to Josie as she left the last sing-a-long rang in Josie's ears and stuck in her brain for days. Josie and Jake Winters had come home from the Pear Blossom sing-along like they were living in two different worlds, and, in fact, they were. Jake came home laughing and clapping and bubbling over as he told his mom how he sang "Twinkle, Twinkle Little Star," and about the lady named Cat who liked him. Every day for a week he asked when he could go back and sing again, and then he seemed to forget about it. He had such a simple life with no real worries of his own.

Josie, on the other hand, was more subdued than usual. "It was fine," she sadly muttered, and that was all she said when Gloria asked her how it went. Josie and her mother were very close, and Josie kept very few things from her mom, so that was an unusually quiet response. Gloria didn't pry, but she worried. Had Jake embarrassed her?

She doubted that, because Josie just did not allow herself to be embarrassed by him. She wondered what had gone wrong, but she knew that when Josie was ready—when she'd thought it all out and was ready to share, they'd discuss whatever had happened.

Josie was different than most 17 year-old girls. Gloria and Mark, Josie's parents, had known for years that just as Jake was special in his own way with Down Syndrome, Josie was unique with her compassionate heart and

her inquisitive mind in wanting to know what made people tick. She'd been reared in a Christian home with two loving parents and with Jake, a very special little brother, whom Josie loved with all her heart. Even before Jake was born, she had an empathetic compassionate heart and a gift for looking past the outward appearance and into the heart of everyone she met. Jake's problem's made her even more tender-hearted and inquisitive about people and their problems. Some people said, "She'll be a psychiatrist when she grows up." "Or a missionary," others whispered.

"She's so precocious!"

"Why does Mrs. Barbour, the neighbor lady, wear those thick, dark glasses summer and winter in sunshine or cloudy days? Is she hiding behind them?" Why? Why? Why? The questions that most three year-olds begin asking never stopped; they just got deeper.

Josie was never rude enough to question people about their actions to their faces, but she'd ponder for hours, and wonder what she could do to help.

Gloria had told her over and over. "You just have to accept people as they are," and "You can't change the whole world, Josie."

Josie's comeback lately had been, "But maybe one person at a time."

Josie had attended public school until she was in the seventh grade. From what she had heard and seen of junior high, she knew she wanted no part of that scene, and so she begged her parents to either home-school her or let her go to a Christian school. Her parents both thought she needed the companionship and extra-curricular activities that a classroom and school setting offered, so after deliberating over their budget and encouraging Josie to help them cut back on expenses, they enrolled her in The Lighthouse Christian Academy in Middleford. She blossomed there into a beautiful, delicate flower. Her roots were strong and as she went through junior high and into high school, her beliefs and her morals were sturdy stems to hold her upright. She wouldn't give in to being whipped by the winds of change in every direction, even in a Christian school. She had made up her mind that her walk of life would follow the path of helping others. Naturally, her friends thought she would work with special needs children. She had often helped with Special Olympic events, and she certainly wouldn't rule that out, but ever since she had been playing the organ at the retirement home, she had seen another spectrum of life, those nearing the end of life, and she decided they had special needs, too. *If I could just see into their hearts,* she thought, *I know I could help them!*

"She doesn't even like herself, Mom! That's what Sarah said about Bertha. Isn't that sad? I think even Jake likes himself!" Sarah finally unloaded her heartache to her mother after brooding about it for almost a week. She had made up her mind what she wanted to do before she cracked open her heart to her mom. Her compassion spilled out and ran down the length of the dining room table where Gloria was seated at the other end.

"Which one is Bertha? What is so special about her?" Gloria asked.

"Well, first of all, she's in a wheel chair. I don't know why or how long she's been in it, but she sure is an unhappy lady! I want to talk with her and find out about her life and see what has made her so bitter, and then there's Essie, and she cries a lot. Why, I don't know. And then there's . . . ."

"Whoa, slow down, girl. One at a time. Are you sure you want to get so involved in their lives? And how do you think you can help them?" Gloria knew that Josie didn't just make acquaintances and then move on; she would try to analyze each personality and each infirmity and then try to figure out what to do for each one.

"I've been thinking that if it's okay with Mrs. Landers I could maybe do my senior project on some of the people I've met at Pear Blossom. Also I would have to talk to the administrator there." Mrs. Landers was Josie's class advisor and the counselor in charge of the senior class projects. She, like everyone else, expected that Josie would do her project on some aspect of Down Syndrome. But Josie was full of surprises. She didn't break the rules or buck authority. She was respectful of her elders, of the rules, and the morals her parents had taught her. Most of all she tried to follow a Godly, Christian life.

But she liked to step out from the crowd, not to be noticed, but to explore avenues that others would never think to walk. She didn't always want to be so predictable. She had learned early on that if she failed she would get up and go on again, and if she didn't try, then that was failure in and of itself.

"So, what do you think, Mom? I haven't worked it all out in my mind yet, but I will. I just want to help these poor, little, old people!"

It didn't really matter what Gloria thought. When Josie's mind was made up, her determination won over any negative ideas Gloria might have, and as long as it was a good and honest idea, Gloria just had to trust God as Josie did, that He would take care of all the details. After all, that was what she and Mark had taught their daughter all along.

Words of admonition did not fall on deaf ears. Josie respected her mother's concerns. She was a mother who cared, and Josie knew that implicitly. So, when Gloria said, "Just be careful, Josie. Plan your work, and work your plan, and do it unto the Lord. But please remember that love is a risk. I know you will come to love these people. Maybe you already do. I just don't want you to be hurt, and you know, some day one of those people will die or move away, and that will be so hard on you." She went to Josie and threw her arms around her. "I am so proud of you, Josie. Let me know how I can help." She knew Josie would need her. There would be tears to wipe away and heartaches to share, but she couldn't help but think that whatever her senior project would entail, it would be a good thing and a blessing in one way or another.

* * *

As Josie predicted, Mrs. Landers was astounded when Josie talked to her the next day about her senior project. "So, this will really be a *senior* project—a senior class student with senior citizens. Are you sure you don't want to do a study on Down Syndrome?"

"That's just it, Mrs. Landers. I've sort of been studying that ever since Jake was born, and I want to do something else for a change. I think old people are so interesting!"

"Well, thanks for the compliment, but please don't call us *old people*! I'm getting there myself, you know. One more year until I retire."

"Oops! Sorry!" Josie blushed a scarlet red. "What should I call them?"

Mrs. Landers ran through the list of titles that senior citizens were called. "In this case, since they live in a retirement home, just call them *residents*. You know, that could be part of your project; find out what they like to be called. You may be surprised by the variety of their answers. There are so many things you can learn from this project. I am getting excited about it myself!" Short, plump Mrs. Landers twisted and turned in her chair, settling in like a hen preparing to lay an egg. "Now, remember, you are still a junior, but it's good to get started early and get a feel for your project. You might even decide it's not what you want to study, and if so, then you have plenty of time before next school year to change your mind. Let me know what the administrator thinks, and if she wants to talk to me about it, she can call. Oh, and be sure to make an appointment first. Don't just pop in."

"Mrs. Landers, this is sort of a hard question to ask you, but I was just wondering . . . do you like yourself?"

Thinking that was an odd question, Mrs. Landers frowned and took her time before she answered. She raised her graying, bushy eyebrows and laughed. "Well, I don't kiss the mirror every time I look in it at myself, but yes, I have a certain sense of dignity and self-respect. I think God has given me certain gifts, and I try to use those for His glory. Why do you ask?"

Josie explained what Sarah had said about Bertha's attitude, and with that, Mrs. Landers could see that Josie didn't just want to get groceries for Bertha and help write a letter.

She'd want to dig deeper. She knew Josie pretty well, and she gave her the same admonition that Sarah's mother had warned. "Just be careful, Josie. You can study them, but you can only help them as far as they want to be helped at this point." She repeated the last three words . . . "at this point . . . this point in their lives, and this point in yours!"

"Got it!" Josie caught the message, but in her heart she knew it would be more than just scratching the surface. She was as determined to try to take apart each resident's problems and heartaches as Jake was to take apart the old alarm clock his daddy had given him. She just hoped she would have more success than he had at putting the pieces back together.

CHAPTER FIFTEEN

The Appointment

"Not as man sees does God see.
Man sees the appearance,
But the Lord looks into the heart.
—I Samuel 16:7

Acting upon the advice of Mrs. Landers, Josie called and made an appointment with Sherrie, the administrator at Pear Blossom. Sherrie thought the meeting was about the sing-a-longs, so she was surprised when Josie said, "No, it's about my senior project."

Wanting to sound professional, Sherrie stifled jokes that bubbled in her mind. She instantly thought that, yes, the residents were all senior projects with their senior moments, but instead she was very business-like, and after asking Josie several questions, she agreed to meet with her at 4:00 p.m. the next day. Actually, Sherrie had no idea what a senior project was since when she had graduated ten years ago, they were not required.

The lobby was unusually quiet when Josie arrived the next afternoon. The mail had come, so the regulars were sequestered away reading their seed catalogs or self-diagnosing their ailments in the latest medical pamphlet they had ordered for two dollars from Dr. Gott.

Essie had just received her information regarding prostate problems. "You know, I have all the symptoms of an enlarged prostate," she had written on her order form to Dr. Gott several weeks before. She was so surprised to read a footnote on the pamphlet that had come.

"Judging from your name, Essie, I assume you are a female, and you do not have the male equipment to have prostate problems. Enclosed is the information you requested."

Dr. Gott had signed it himself.

"But I have all the symptoms," Essie said right out loud to the pamphlet.

Bertha was perusing the Burpee's Seed catalog. She hoped her name would be drawn for a garden box out on the east side of the building. There were only ten wooden boxes, so that was very limiting. Her name had never been drawn, but last year Winnie had shared hers with her. Winnie lost interest after the first weed appeared, so Bertha ended up with the work and the bounty. It was amazing what two tomato plants could produce.

Gayle had planted one zucchini plant, which overran the box, trailed on the cement, and riled up the other gardeners until it began producing, and then when she had enough zucchini for the whole establishment, she was popular again. "I feel like a mother," she beamed, as she lovingly caressed the long, green vegetables, "and from the looks of them, they are all boys!"

Pastor Paul Clairmont was the only resident that was still in the lobby after mail-call.

The soft cushions of the couch nearly swallowed up his short, plump body, and he looked over his reading glasses when he heard the automatic door swing open.

"Josie? Josie Winters?" His deep voice caught Josie off guard. She had known Pastor Paul all of her life. In fact, he had baptized her several years before, and then when he retired, she had lost track of him. She had no idea what he was doing at Pear Blossom.

Glancing quickly at her watch, she was assured that she had a couple minutes to visit with him. "What are you doing here?" They said to each other at the exact same time, and then they both laughed. She had always loved his deep belly laugh, and the way his tummy jiggled like Santa Claus.

"You aren't old enough to be here," he said, as he struggled to his feet to politely stand in the presence of a young lady. "Here, sit down, and we'll talk." He reminded Josie of the plump dumplings her mother arranged on top of the chicken and noodles.

Josie had never seen him at the sing-a-longs, and when she told him she and Jake had recently entertained in the Community Room, he was surprised. "Well, if I'd have realized it was you, I would have been there." He promised to watch the bulletin board and come next time. He answered Josie's question of what he was doing there by explaining that since his wife had passed two years ago, he didn't want the house any more, so he had moved in here. "It's hard to completely retire from the ministry, so I lead a Bible study here, and try to be a witness without being too pushy. Sort of like your dad, Josie. 'Once a Marine, always a Marine.' 'Once a pastor, always a pastor.'" He smoothed his neatly groomed white moustache.

Josie had just started telling Pastor Paul why she was there when Sherrie popped out of her office and motioned for her to come in for their meeting.

"I want to hear more about this senior project, Josie. Maybe I can help you somehow with the details." That was the one attribute that Josie remembered the most about him—his willingness to always be available to lend a hand or give advice in a professional but loving way.

Josie assured him that she would contact him, and as he handed her his business card, he added, "Just call the number on here, and we can meet over there." He waved his hand in the direction of the library. "So good to see you again, Josie." He stood again as Josie arose and waved good-bye and disappeared into Sherrie's office.

"Do you know Pastor Paul?" Sherrie quizzed Josie, as she showed her to a chair across from her desk.

"Oh, just for all of my life. I haven't seen him for awhile, and he sure has aged . . . I mean he looks more like a grandfather . . . I mean . . ."

"That's okay, Josie. You didn't really say anything wrong. Sometimes these people seem to age overnight. Just don't let them hear you say it. They are trying so hard to stay young even though sometimes some of them act like they are in their second childhood. Anyway, what's this senior project all about?"

Josie explained in detail: 40 hours of volunteering, 20 page paper, Power Point presentation and a fifteen minute speech in front of judges at school. "And my advisor has to sign-off on my ideas and progress as I go along, so I have to take notes and meet with her a couple times a month." Josie was pretty sure she would have more than 20 hours at Pear Blossom; she had so much to do and she didn't even know where to start. "That's why I'm here. I need your approval and ideas of what the residents need me to do."

Sherrie was overwhelmed with Josie's determination, and she could see her compassion written on her sleeve. She needed some time to think. This was a new predicament. She'd spent the morning doing the usual paperwork, showing a prospective resident an apartment, and checking on Maria, whose daughter had called with a worried tone to her voice concerning Maria's depression. She'd never had to help map out a student's senior project whose grade point average and graduation depended somewhat on Sherrie's planning. This was not in her job description!

Finally, after getting Josie a Coke from the little refrigerator in the back of her office, she suggested that Josie attend the next Association meeting to get a glimpse into upcoming events that the residents might be planning, and to meet with Betty, the Activities Director

"Oh, and the library needs some work."

Josie agreed to that, but she wanted more than to just deal with events and rearrange books. She wanted to help Bertha to like herself and to cheer up Essie, so she wouldn't cry any more.

CHAPTER SIXTEEN

The Association Meeting

"I won't insult your intelligence by
suggesting that you really believe
what you said."
—William F. Buckley, Jr.

The monthly meeting of The Association of Residents was scheduled to start *promptly* at 7:00 p.m., as the notification had stated. Bertha was on the peck before the meeting ever was actually called to order because of the stragglers who showed up a couple minutes after. She had stated at every single meeting that if the *strays* missed roll call, then they had no right to vote on any of the issues, and at every single meeting, Duke, the new president of the group, had just shaken his head in disbelief and told her that, "We just can't be that strict with our rules, Bertha," to which she retorted, "Well, if they really cared about what goes on here like I do, they'd be here on time." She always sat in the back by the door, so she could monitor their arrivals, since Duke wouldn't close the doors after 7:00 as she had suggested.

Sarah had begged and coaxed and bribed Maria with another mocha to get her to come. "Just try it just this once, and then you'll know what to expect in the way of activities and what is coming up in the spring." Maria finally reluctantly conceded, more to appease Sarah than any great desire to leave her apartment and get involved. Since Maria was always prompt, if not early for appointments, it was no problem getting there on time, and Sarah was thankful for that. Maria's first meeting would be her last if Bertha chastised her as she came in the door.

"What is that you are drinking?" Bertha scowled at Maria. "We don't allow food or drinks at these meetings."

Sarah gently extricated the plastic cup from Maria's fingers and placed it in the receptacle nearby. "She was just finishing up, Bertha."

Maria was ready to cut and run because it was the caffeine high that had gotten her there in the first place, but Sarah placed her hand at her elbow and escorted her to a seat.

"It's pretty hard to ignore her, but we have to try. Don't take it personally. I'll get you another mocha tomorrow," she assured Maria, who was looking fearfully around the room to see who was next to pounce on her.

"I shouldn't have come," Maria's voice quavered. "It's just too soon. I'm not ready for this. If I felt better, I'd hold my own against that woman, but I'm overcome with weakness."

Sarah and Betty had spent the week since Cat left trying to cheer up Maria. They'd checked on her every morning and made suggestions for the day, as their time allowed, but she always had an excuse for staying home.

"She is acting almost like someone died," Betty had worried to Sarah that afternoon.

"Well, Cat told me that she does suffer from depression, and as we all know, it is a big adjustment separating from the old life. Almost like a burial. Burying the past and trying to go on. It was a lot easier to move around when we were younger, Betty, and she told me this is her last move, which sounds so final. Oh, but one positive thing that happened is that Michael and Jillian—you know, her son, had her over to their house for dinner on Sunday."

Betty was relieved to hear that she had spent some time with family. "I think she will fit right in here, if she will just try. Maybe I can talk her into helping with the activities."

The Community Room filled with residents, and by 7:00 p.m. almost every seat was taken. Duke was pleased to see such a good crowd, but spring always did that. People got out more and mingled, even if just amongst themselves in the building, and they were eager for outside activities, spring cleaning, and fresh air, all of which were on the agenda for the night.

Who should come in late to the meeting, but the administrator? Bertha was beside herself and pointed to her watch and glared at Sherrie. If that wasn't bad enough for Bertha's blood pressure, she had that girl with her who played the organ! And, to top it all off, Sherrie was trying to sneak in the door with a soda! At least Josie didn't have that Mongoloid with her.

"What is that you are drinking? This is a business meeting, not a social hour." Bertha reprimanded Sherrie, and she didn't care who heard her. "No intelligence whatsoever!"

Of course, Millie couldn't hear. "What did she say?" Millie said in her stage whisper that was heard all over the room. "Did she say *shrinking?*"

Sherrie knew that the Community Room had no rules about eating or drinking, so she tried to politely ignore Bertha, and she and Josie took a seat by Maria. Now, if Sherrie would have walked into the library with a beverage, Bertha would have had some ground on which to stand. That was the one room where food and drinks were outlawed, although Essie had taken popcorn and sandwiches in for late night snacks, had gotten caught and tried to hide the evidence under the cushions. Betty had been the private eye on that infraction, but she spoke quietly and personally to Essie about it, and it apparently had never happened again.

The meeting began, and Josie noticed right away that they did not follow Robert's Rules of Order. Bertha had all but given up on teaching the group correct parliamentary procedure, so she sat in the back and made notes on her yellow legal pad. She'd straighten Duke out later.

The minutes of the last meeting were read, but never approved. A motion was made and seconded, but never voted on. Bertha kept yelling, "Question. I'm calling for the question."

"We don't have any questions!" Betty yelled back, and so the meeting went on.

When they finally got to New Business, the meeting picked up steam.

Duke announced that the first order of New Business was to draw for the garden boxes. The pre-registration had been completed before the meeting, but there were always a few who had forgotten to put their name in the box.

"It's too late now," Bertha reminded them. "If your name is not in the box, then don't be disappointed when they don't draw your name. It's your own fault."

Sherrie suggested that Josie draw the ten names. That way surely it would be deemed fair to Bertha. She drew several names, and each resident was thrilled to be chosen and began to have visions of flowers or vegetables. "Number 8 is Maria!" Sarah and Betty both clapped when they heard Josie call her name. Betty had talked her into registering.

"But who will help me with it?" Maria made worry an art form, and she was already to paint a dismal picture. "You know, I don't see too well." Sarah and Betty calmed her down with their offers of assistance.

Sherrie had an *ah ha* moment. "Josie can help you," she whispered in Maria's ear. "She's going to be coming around here more and helping out. A school project." Sherrie nodded and smiled at Maria, hoping that would cheer her up a bit.

Josie had drawn another name—Emily—one of the sweetest little ladies in the whole place. She lived upstairs in 301 and rarely got involved in the back-stabbing and politics of Pear Blossom. "We see enough of that on the telly," she always said, when asked to hold an office, but she did like to garden, so she had applied.

"And the last name is . . . drum roll! . . . Blanche"

Oh, the Bird Woman! Maria couldn't wait to tell Cat. She could picture her pulling a long worm out of the ground and pecking through the dirt looking for stray seeds.

Bertha was in shock! If she could have done the impossible and jumped up from her wheel chair, that would have been the time! But instead she had to settle for frowning and glaring and grumbling. There must have been a mistake. Perhaps her name somehow got stuck to the side of the box and wasn't in the proper position for drawing. She'd check the box afterwards, and she did, only to find that her name was nowhere to be seen. Sabotage!

For the third year in a row, her name was not drawn, and now this. She had actually forgotten to enter her name this year, but, of course, that option was not possible. Bertha prided herself on her memory, so it had to be dirty, underhanded sabotage! "I'm surprised I don't die of apoplexy," she muttered to Winnie, whose name hadn't appeared either, but she didn't really care.

The New Business continued with the next order being the Spring Garage Sale. Millie, who had wanted a boutique year-round, had volunteered to step into the position of chairman, as long as she could change the name from *garage sale* to something else. "It's so ridiculous when we don't have garages!" Her idea had met with resounding approval, but for want of a better name, she had come up with the temporary term, *Yard Sale*.

Other names were thrown out and bandied about—*Spring Cleaning Sale, Inside Yard Sale, Dollar Sale,* and *Pre-Boutique Sale.* The final vote was 20 to 4, in favor of *Spring Cleaning Sale.* Bertha abstained, stating that nobody would know what that meant. Millie suggested that under the big lettering, the words *Yard Sale* could be written in, so Bertha was somewhat appeased.

The date was set for the weekend of March 20 and 21, although some protested that it was so far into the month that the Social Security checks would have been spent and nobody would have any money left for shopping.

"Learn to budget," Sarah threw out that idea, knowing that it was too late for most of them to learn anything new or change their ways.

"How can I budget when it's already all spoken for?" Winnie blurted out from the back row. Betty had an ideal answer regarding Winnie's spending with her drinking habit, but curbed her tongue.

Millie assured everyone that she would be contacting them for help. She passed around a sign-up sheet for tables, and Betty volunteered to help Duke with advertising. "We have those big sandwich boards that Chester made—God rest his soul—, so we'll need a man to volunteer to help Duke set those up down on the corner the morning of the sale." Emily thought maybe she could volunteer her male friend, Herb, but she told Betty she would have to check with him. She was eager to sign up for a table to sell Avon, as she had a lot of Christmas items left over—all marked down, of course.

The last order of New Business was for involvement in the annual Pear Blossom Festival, which was scheduled for April 7 and 8. The whole town of Middleford was involved with everything from a parade, a fun run, a pet show, an art show, to a barbeque and more.

A few of the residents participated in the local, yearly event. Sarah always helped with The Friends of the Library Book Sale and Quilt Raffle drawing, and Oscar would have a watercolor painting on display at the Ann Miller Theater. "My *hanging*," he secretly told Millie.

Antonio entered the chili cook-off every year. Last year he earned first place, and his prize was a year's supply of chili powder. "That's what the certificate read, but who would ever be able to judge how much a year's supply would be? Wouldn't it vary from one cook to another?" Bertha argued. "What a waste!"

Maria perked up when she heard the word *April.* "That's when Cat comes," she whispered to Sarah and Betty. "So I'll be busy!" She hoped that would be true.

Nothing was decided as far as the facility's involvement as a whole in the festival. "If we had a van or a float to ride on," they lamented, "we could be in the parade." Betty announced that, "I'll leave my door open to suggestions and if anyone gets a brilliant idea, let me know."

Josie's mind was working on all cylinders. There's that old float in the school bus garage. If we could just re-decorate it . . . maybe . . . , but she just let the idea simmer for the time being. She'd mention it to Sherrie later.

Thinking the meeting was over, the buzzing of conversation began, and Duke had to bang his gavel for attention. Maria jumped, as she had momentarily dozed off, and Winnie was getting antsy and needing to pop the cork on her cane.

"What did he say?" Millie asked, getting right up in Essie's face. "Did he say *boutique?*"

"Meeting adjourned!" Bertha bellowed, echoing what Duke had already announced over the humming of the busy bees.

The chatter continued, and although it was getting on into the evening, it was a good time to socialize for a few minutes. Bertha wheeled up the aisle to catch Duke and educate him on a few pointers. She could not tolerate his ignorance of procedures.

Meanwhile, an admirer had been decorating Maria's door once again.

CHAPTER SEVENTEEN

Maria's Admirer

"And now in age, I bud again.
                    —George Herbert

"What's new?" Josie asked Essie, as they left the meeting and ambled into the lobby.

"Oh, I'm too old to have anything new," Essie said, as she patted Josie on the back. "By the way, it's nice to see you. How is your little brother? Is he coming to sing again?"

"Oh, maybe someday. He wants to come every time, I think, but my mom won't let him. But I'm going to be here a lot more doing my Senior Project."

"What is that, dear? Are we projects? I know some of us are tough nuts to crack—like Bertha! That's for sure." Essie grimaced and shook her head.

Josie explained a little of what it was all about, but she told Essie she needed to talk to Sherrie and plan it all out before she got too involved, but she assured Essie she would include her in her project and Bertha, too.

"Well, good luck working with her. You'll need it! She thinks she knows everything, but she doesn't. I get up at all hours of the night, and I know what goes on then, and she is clueless. Why, just last night, I looked out the window and guess what I saw?" She was suddenly interrupted by Gayle's barking dog.

"She has to go right now!" Gayle said, as she hurried the little ball of fur off the elevator.

"Did she say she has vertigo?" Millie wondered, as she appeared out of nowhere. "I had it when I was auditioning for *Oklahoma*. Of course, I didn't get the part. How could I with all that dancing and spinning around when my head was already spinning? You can imagine how disappointed I was," Millie pouted, thinking back over her lost role.

"There's another project for you," Essie said wisely and pointed at Millie, as they were nearing the office door. Sherrie was waiting for a short discussion with Josie about the evening meeting, so Essie went on her way.

Winnie had stumped down the hallway quickly. She needed a drink! The procession that followed Winnie to escort Maria back to her apartment consisted of Betty and Sarah.

"Oh, you don't need to see me home, girls. I am fine," Maria protested to no avail. "But I do love a parade!" She stifled a laugh, not wanting them to think her depression was over. She was enjoying the attention and companionship, and she felt that she could develop a real genuine friendship with these two.

They had arrived at Maria's apartment. "What is that?" Sarah was the first to notice a basket on the floor in front of the door.

"Oh, it's some spring flowers. Yellow tulips and daffy dills!" Betty chimed in.

"Can someone pick it up for me?" Maria asked. "My back is so stiff from sitting on those hard chairs at the meeting."

"Not me!" Sarah waved them away, as Betty obliged. "I have allergies, you know."

"I bet it's from Jillian. Oh, I hope she and Michael weren't here while I was out. Betty, can you read the card for me?" By now, they were in Maria's kitchen, and she had flipped on the overhead light. Sarah kept her distance. No need to borrow trouble and start sneezing.

"A touch of spring for a lovely lady." And it was signed, "P.C."

"Who in the world?" Maria was astonished once again. Not one of the three had a clue. They ruled out all the likely suspects in the building—Antonio, Oscar, and Otis. Even Tony was scrutinized under their mental microscopes to no avail.

"Well, I must get home." Sarah was edging toward the door, "but I'll sleep on it. You know, I do my best thinking in the middle of the night when I am trying to forget about the hot flashes, or when I am in the bathroom for long periods."

Periods? Maria thought, oh, surely not at her age! But she let it go.

"Call me, girls, if you figure it out, but not in the middle of the night!" And Maria waved them out the door. She was so exhausted. "I'll worry about you tomorrow," she told the tulips.

That, of course, was exactly when Sarah figured it out. Around 2:45 a.m., after answering Mother Nature's second call of the night, Sarah was having a terrible time getting back to sleep. Counting sheep never worked and neither did praying. That only brought to mind all her friends and their problems and worried her into a state of nerves and jitters, and then she was awake until dawn was about to crack open her golden egg. She did love puzzles, though, and those letters, P.C., were a real enigma. Her mind wandered up one corridor and down another. She pretty much knew everyone in the building and where they lived, except for the new lady named Blanche, the *bird lady.*

Sarah's mind stopped outside every door and took a quick inventory of the inhabitants inside. When she had almost given up, that's when it came to her! Isn't that just the way it always happens? She had forgotten to let her mind travel down past Bertha's door and the laundry room to those other apartments on the west side. P.C, why, you old codger you! Sarah couldn't believe her own thoughts. But it must be! He is the only one with those initials! She rolled over and smiled and was so pleased with herself. She couldn't wait until a reasonable hour to call Maria and tell her the news! At least he was a nice man. Maria was lucky. No, not lucky; she was blessed!

Eight, nine, nine-thirty. The minutes ticked off, and Sarah didn't know when to call Maria. Finally, at 9:45 she could wait no longer.

"Oh, hello, Maria, did I wake you up?" She didn't wait for Maria's answer, and frankly she didn't care if she had at that point. "I got it! I figured it out! I hope you like mustaches."

"Well, I'm not going to kiss him, whoever it is!" Maria thought this had gone far enough. "So, who is P.C.?"

"Paul Clairmont! It has to be! It just has to be!" Sarah sounded as excited as if she had won the Oregon State Lottery, but Maria had no idea who in the world Paul Clairmont was.

"Don't you remember him? He gave the blessing at the potluck. He is a retired pastor."

Maria didn't believe her and barely remembered him. "Sarah, do you think a pastor would be sending Valentines and poems and flowers? Besides, he doesn't even know me! My stars! The men sure work fast around here. I've never seen the likes of it," Maria was in shock.

Sarah was sure it had to be Pastor Paul. "He is lonely, I know that. His wife died two years ago, and he sold their house, and moved in here. I'm sure you've seen him. He sits in the corner chair in the lobby and usually has a book in his hand. I have seen him, though, many times looking over the book and watching what is going on, so I s'pose he has been observing you, too. Oh, isn't that romantic, Maria?"

"Well, I suppose it could be if I was younger. I didn't move in here to look for romance or to find a man. Lord knows, I've had enough of that to last a lifetime. I wonder if he gives others in here gifts and poems, and remember, Sarah, some of those were from Tony for Cat."

"Maybe he'll ask you to church or to come to Bible study. Oh, isn't this exciting?"

"Oh, I just don't know what to think. I have always been a Presbyterian, but I haven't been in a church in years, except for Michael's wedding, and that was in a Lutheran church. I wouldn't know how to act. I'll have to discuss this with Cat. Oh, well, he hasn't asked me yet. I've never even talked to him. I think we are getting ahead of ourselves here, Sarah, especially if he's a Baptist."

But they weren't. Later that day when Maria went out in front to sit on the bench to enjoy some sunshine for a few minutes, she soon saw the doors swing open and a figure approach the bench. With the glare of the sun and her failing eyesight, she couldn't see the person's face, but the deep voice gave away his gender. She knew immediately that she should have stayed inside. She didn't feel like having to carry on a conversation with anyone, let alone a man. Sunshine helped her depression, but she was still swimming upstream.

"A beautiful day, isn't it?" The voice dripped with smooth honey. "Do you mind if I sit here and let it warm my face? Oh, where are my manners?" he continued, as he sat down uninvited. "I don't believe we have met. I am Pastor Paul Clairmont."

Maria could see that he was holding out his hand, and so she shook it, germs and all. She wiggled around on the cushion on the bench and tried to see his face. "Oh, yes, I remember. Didn't you pray for the food at the potluck? Oh, I mean you asked the blessing." She had already embarrassed herself and with a Baptist!

Paul, though, thought it was an appropriate way to state it. "You know, sometimes I do think I should pray for the food; we never know what we might be getting at those potlucks." His laughter shook the whole bench. "Sometimes I just ask the blessing and then leave."

Maria wondered if he had stayed and eaten some of her cannelloni, but she didn't want to ask.

She didn't have to. He filled in the blanks himself with his soothing, sonorous voice. "I did stay the other night, though, and I'm sure glad I did. Someone brought the best Italian dish. Did you have any of it? My, it was good! In fact, I went back for a second helping." Actually, he had seen her bring it in, but she didn't need to know all his secrets.

"Yes, it did turn out quite good this time. My daughter helped me make it. It's one of my family's recipes from Italy." Oops, too much information, Maria thought, and so soon.

"Oh, you're Italian?" Pastor Paul acted surprised. Maria looked it and talked it with her hands, he had noticed. "I'm just a short, dumpy Heinz 57 Varieties myself." Then he realized that Maria was short and square, too. "Someone told me that I am just short for my weight. Isn't that a good one?" He hoped she would agree, and she laughed out loud for the first time in days.

Their conversation continued, and other residents came and went. The only one who paid any attention to them was Sarah, who came out to wait for Jess. She could hardly contain herself when she saw the two of them together.

"Oh, hello, you two. I see that you've met." She planted herself squarely in front of them.

Maria hoped that Sarah would control herself and not blurt out any unnecessary information that Pastor Paul could live without hearing. Fortunately, all she offered was the weather report, which they'd already covered. And then Jess came and whisked her away.

"Now, there's a sweet lady," Pastor Paul said. 'She's been coming to our Wednesday afternoon Bible study in the library. She always has a story to tell."

"I bet she does," Maria could certainly agree with him on that score. "She is a nice lady, but she seems to have a lot of physical problems."

"Well, just look around this place. We all do. She just gives more organ recitals than most of us." He laughed at his own joke, and the bench shook once more.

Maria decided she'd had enough hilarity and sunshine for one day, so she began to excuse herself, and she struggled to her feet. Pastor Paul wanted to help her up from the bench, but his arthritis slowed him down.

"One more thing before you go, Maria," Paul grabbed her arm, as he struggled to his feet. "I wanted to personally invite you to Bible study on Wednesday. You know, it meets right next door to your apartment in the library."

So, he does know where I live, she thought. "But I'm not a Baptist!" Maria decided to inform him of her religious persuasion. "I've been a Presbyterian since I was a little girl."

"That doesn't matter. We just study the personal relationship of God's word."

Personal relationship? Ah, ha! That's what I thought you wanted, she thought as they entered the lobby. She took it . . . well, personally, when that wasn't exactly what he meant.

He wanted to ask her if she liked the flowers, and she wanted to ask if he was the one who had been bearing gifts, but their questions got caught in the closing of the big, glass front doors, and once they entered the lobby, there was Bertha, who had been watching out the window the whole time.

His parting words to Maria raised Bertha's eyebrows and dangled question marks in front of her thick glasses. "I hope you decide to come, Maria, and find new life. You know, the highways are littered with flat squirrels who couldn't make up their minds."

"What a thing to say to me!" Maria told Sarah later in the day. "I liked him at first, but then, all of a sudden, I didn't know what he was talking about. What do flat squirrels have to do with anything?"

Sarah tried to explain his sense of humor and his colorful way of speaking to Maria. "I just think he was trying to find a way to get you to come to Bible study. Pastors have their own little object lessons and sayings, and have you ever noticed how sometimes they like to start off their sermons with a joke? I always thought that was odd, but then I decided that God must have a sense of humor, too. Just look around at all the funny people He created."

"Yeah, mixed nuts!"

"Oh, that's a good one, Maria. I bet Pastor Paul would like that and could use it in his lessons. You'll just have to come next Wednesday." Sarah's words of encouragement only added more turmoil to Maria's undecided mind. "By the way, have you told Cat yet about P.C.?"

Maria had called Cat that morning as soon as she had talked to Sarah. "Yes, and was she ever surprised! She thought those letters stood for *personal computer* or *politically correct*. When she found out it was a pastor, she laughed and laughed because she suspected either Antonio or Otis or Oscar as being sweet on me."

"I guess you brought some humor into her life, then, Maria. That is good!"

Maria rebounded by saying that Cat's life had been anything but dull and boring. "She said she hears from Tony every day, and she found a publisher for her book—you know, the one she is writing about a retirement home."

RESIDENT'S BULLETIN BOARD

DATE: MARCH 10, 2007
MEMO: TO ALL PEAR BLOSSOM RESIDENTS:
FROM   SHERRIE, THE ADMINISTRATOR:
RE: DISAPPEARING ITEMS

It has been brought to my attention recently that several items have disappeared, and they need to be returned to their proper owners. Last night a wind chime was taken from beside the door of a resident's apartment. This was a very special Valentine gift to the resident, and she would really like it back. In February, the decorations that were on the windowsill of the third floor were taken. Also the newspaper that is donated to be read in the library is starting to disappear again before the day is through. The newspaper needs to remain in the lounge until Sarah picks it up at 7:00 p.m.

The "freebie" table in the Community Room is the first table on the left as you come in the door. This is the only place where free items are left and can be taken. If you see other stray items lying around the facility, please bring them to the office so that we can find the owner. Don't just take the items assuming they are free.

Probably the greatest problem occurred over the weekend in the laundry. Someone took some sheets out of a washing machine, and they were still wet! The owner was terribly upset!

If you have seen any of these items, please bring them down to the office, and no questions will be asked. Please dry the sheets first.

Thank you for your time in searching for these missing items.

>>>>>>>>>>>>>>>>>>>>

FOR SALE!!!!

COFFEE TABLE: 4 feet x 1 and ½ feet Legs to be screwed in, but the screws don't fit. (It was a bad buy at Howard's sale). Does anybody have an idea how I can get rid of this big, heavy piece of wood? View it now at Blanche's in Apt. 206.

TWO CEMETERY LOTS FOR SALE: Call Winnie 659 0099

CHAPTER EIGHTEEN

Spring Cleaning Sale

Frosts are slain and flowers begotten,
And in green underwood and cover
Blossom by blossom the spring begins.
—Swinburne

Spring came roaring through Middleford like the waters of Bear Creek that rises and yells "Flood" from the top of her lungs. Bear Creek rarely keeps her promise, and the city remains dry, but there is always that vengeful spirit that some day she just might call for high-water pants and sandbags, and let her true feelings wash over the town.

But in March of 2007 Bear Creek was calm. The mild winter shrugged her shoulders and threw off her coat and decided she had failed at snowstorms and rain, so she whooshed into town dressed up like spring with heat and insects and dust.

Pear Blossom Plaza received a good springtime bath inside and out. Tony hosed down the entire building on the outside and washed the windows inside and out. The tongue-waggers in the lobby thought that the huge blinds over the front window looked dirty, and as they were wondering how Tony could clean them, Winnie stomped into the scene just in time to come to their rescue. "Why don't you wash them from the outside?" Winnie wisely stated, as she shook her cane at the window.

The five women involved in the discussion looked from one to another, frowning in wonderment of just how that would work. They rested their jaws in their hands and shook their heads and frowned some more, and they finally all decided about the same time that Winnie's answer was for the birds.

"What did she say? Wash them from the outside?" Millie had heard correctly for once. "Why, that wouldn't work, Winnie. What were you thinking?" Millie handled her with kid gloves. "I think you are a little mixed up," Millie sweetly advised her, slipping into her actress role. "Speaking of windows, did you know that I tried out for a part in *Rear Window*?"

Winnie ignored her and wondered what the difference was—"Inside? Outside? Front or rear? Who cares? I was just trying to help," she grumbled, and off she went down the hallway toward Bertha's apartment.

"I must be going, too," the Bird Woman chirped, as she pushed the grocery cart toward the door. "I have to sort through things for the Spring Cleaning Sale, and it's a long ways to walk to the storage unit, and then back," she added. No one could take her because of the cart. "Just make sure I get home before dark," she alerted the other nesters.

Betty agreed to watch for her return later on in the afternoon. "We look out for one another here, Blanche," Betty reassured the Bird Woman, who clapped her hands in delight.

"It's good to feel safe once again," Blanche rubbed her skinny arms where the bruises her son had inflicted had finally faded. "I need you all!" she said, as she pushed the cart out the door. She felt love and trust from these similar souls. She didn't know what each had endured in his or her lifetime, but she felt she wasn't the only one bearing scars and feeling pain.

What she met up with, though, at the storage unit, sent her reeling back to the past and broke her heart again. The strong smell of liquor smacked her in the face as she unlocked the door and pushed the cart onto the cement floor. Empty beer cans littered the floor, and a Jim Beam bottle had her favorite plastic flower arrangement stuck in its neck. Someone had looted the place, and there was nothing of any value left. She didn't have much to begin with, but now she didn't even have anything to sell.

"Oh, I hope they didn't get into my old trunk," she whispered to a little, gray mouse who was stuck in a mouse trap. The dead, beady eyes looked right through her, as if to say, "I know who did it, but they killed me so I wouldn't squeal."

The Bird Woman abandoned the cart just inside the door, and kicking cans aside, she made her way to where she had stored her old, black trunk with the gold handles and lock. Her worst fears were true; the lock was broken, and the trunk had been opened. Glass picture frames were smashed into jagged pieces, and her wedding picture was ripped in half. The words, "Gotcha, Grannie—Good-bye forever," had been sloppily printed in red lipstick on her marriage license of 1935. She recognized that old tube of lipstick. It was nearly dried up now but had been her favorite color.

She reached up in the gray lining of the lid of the trunk where the secret compartment hid her greatest treasure, her late father's coin collection that nobody knew she owned. It was sewn shut with big hemming stitches that matched the lining, and as she pulled the stitches open, she could feel the old familiar cardboard squares of mounted coins. Each one was still encased in plastic, and her sigh of relief could have almost revived that dead, gray mouse. Now all she had to do was get them out and hide them in her clothing and get them home to Pear Blossom. She was thankful she had worn her trench coat with the big pockets. It was the only wind-breaker coat she owned, and it was perfect for the blustery March days.

Looking furtively around the storage unit as if she could feel a thousand eyes watching her, she removed the cardboard casings of coins and tucked them into the big pockets of her coat.

When she could feel no more treasures hidden in the lining, she slammed down the top of the trunk. The contract for the storage unit was in her grandson's name, so she had no reason to come back here again. A broken, empty trunk had no meaning to her, and so she closed another door of her life. She didn't even bother to secure the lock.

"My ace in the hole," she whispered to the mouse, who still stared straight ahead. She patted her pockets, grabbed the empty grocery cart, and made her way as quickly as she could back to Pear Blossom Plaza. Every car that back-fired and every horn that honked made her wish she really was a bird and could fly home to her nest, but she made it safely and long before Betty had started watching for her. She was glad the lobby was deserted, so she didn't have to explain her empty cart. She put it away in the closet of the Community Room, and that too was another chapter ending; she wouldn't be using the cart again.

Betty was just entering the lobby as the Bird Woman returned from the Community Room, and Betty was surprised to see her so soon.

"It was easy to finish up there, and I found what I wanted," she assured Betty that all was well, and she tried to pat her pockets inconspicuously. She was anxious to get to her apartment and put her treasure away. She'd just have to find a few things around her apartment for the Spring Cleaning Sale, which was what several of the residents had been doing all day. But first she had to find a safe hiding place for her coins. Her father had buried them in two coffee cans in his back yard. When he passed away, she found a note and a little map drawn in pencil. She was to have the coins, and his directions showed her just where to look.

"Well, I don't have any coffee cans, and I don't have a back yard, so that's out. Guess I will put you in the freezer. Putting you under the mattress is too obvious; everyone does that," she said to her treasures, as she placed them carefully in a plastic grocery sack from the Grocery outlet. "Now you'll be safe," she continued talking to her coins as she placed the grocery bag behind a loaf of bread and an ice cream carton in her sparsely filled freezer. She still had one key to the storage unit, and Beau had the other. She hoped he wouldn't come looking for it or tell anyone she had it, but she figured he'd just skip out on the contract, and the owners would clean up the place, dispose of the trunk, and rent it out again to someone else. She tossed the key into the freezer, as well, and closed the door on her cold, hard cash.

*   *   *

Maria threw up her hands in despair. Betty, Sarah, and she were discussing the upcoming sale and what wares they had to sell. "I cleaned everything out—Cat helped me—right before I moved. I have nothing to sell! We took oceans of stuff to the Salvation Army Thrift Store, we sold some furniture and my car, and we even gave picture frames to my hairdresser. I couldn't fill a table of items if my life depended on it. Too bad because I sorta wanted to have a sale table," she said sadly.

Betty was a packrat, so she had no trouble weeding out books, videos, knickknacks, and clothes galore. Her problem was that she just hated to part with anything. "The day after I sell it, I'll need it," she vowed, as she picked through her white mop of hair.

"Oh, I know," Sarah agreed. "That always happens to me, too. I am going to sell my meat grinder, though, and those magnets that are in my bed to help my back just have to go. They are as hard as nails, and I've been sleeping in my recliner lately. It is so much more comfortable. I'll find lots more stuff, too. I just know I will."

Meanwhile, Emily was upstairs organizing her Avon collectibles to sell, and Millie was talking to Herb about helping put up the signs. Others were sorting and cleaning and getting items priced for the big sale.

"But who will come?" Maria wondered to her friends.

"People from the outside," Betty answered her. "Oh dear, that sounds like we are imprisoned," she laughed and then went on, "And if nobody comes, we just sell to each other. Sometimes the stuff never leaves the building. Around and around it goes."

By the time the day of the sale came, Maria had a table full of items and no one was the wiser. Betty and Sarah wondered where it all came from, but they were her friends and didn't ask. Jillian wanted to have a sale at her house, but she really didn't have enough to go to all the trouble, so she hauled it into Maria's apartment late at night at the side door. Maria warned her not to bring any children's or men's items, because that would cause question marks and problems. There was a nice array of baskets, dishes, knickknacks, and books, and Maria was proud of her display after all. Later she told Betty and Sarah her little secret, and "Jillian let me keep the money!" That was the best part of all.

Herb called Millie very early Friday morning to announce that he was "down in the back," and he wouldn't be able to put up the signs at the corner and out in front. Millie knew what he meant, but later Essie wondered why he would be "down in the back," or at the garbage can area so early and for so long that he couldn't help as promised. "Why is he dumping or recycling so early? Down in the back?" She couldn't figure it out, and Millie was too busy rounding up Tony to help Duke to answer her questions.

Bertha's table was pitiful! An old rusty bedpan, big black heavily-worn shoes, and a torn shower curtain were the main attractions that she arranged and rearranged several times during the day. "Why do they mess up my table and then not buy anything?" she grumbled to Winnie, who was sharing Bertha's table. Later in the day a man bought her bedpan for his wife for her flower garden. "Can you imagine putting pansies in that? How stupid!" I didn't discourage him, though. A sale's a sale."

Winnie sold some glass bottles and flasks and her old, unadorned cane. The main thing she wanted to get rid of was her television set, and it was on the floor under the table. "I'm getting a new one, and it's plasma," she bragged to everyone in attendance.

"Plasma? Isn't that blood? What's blood got to do with it?" Maria wondered, but nobody could explain it to her.

Millie butted in, "Did she say *love*? Love has to do with everything," and the confusion went on for two days, only to be interrupted by customers.

When Millie wasn't busy with buyers or dragging in more costumes and other articles of clothing, she sat on her table and sang. Her voice was high-pitched and scratchy, like fingernails on the blackboard, but Sarah liked the show tunes. "If I have to hear Jess's classical music and Beethoven's Fifth one more time, I will scream!" Sarah told Maria. "One of my favorites is *Lida Rose* from *The Music Man*. Do you know that one, Millie? We could sing it together."

Yes, Millie did, and with Sarah's alto voice they harmonized and serenaded as folks filtered in and out. "You know, if we practiced some more, we could sing some duets when Josie comes next time for the sing-a-long," Millie said, dying to be back on the stage.

Sarah didn't think too highly of that idea. "We'll see," which was a good pat answer for a lot of unanswerable questions. "With my springtime allergies, I just can't plan ahead."

Pastor Paul Clairmont was one of the late arrivals Saturday afternoon to look over the last of the sale items.

"It's slim pickings, Pastor. You should have been here earlier," Bertha chided him. "We're packing it away for the Goodwill now," she went on, as she threw the big, black shoes in a box.

He politely smiled and glanced her way and could instantly see that she had nothing to suit him. Neither did Millie with her feathery boas and long dresses which swung from a clothesline she had rigged up near the kitchen. He visited with Emily and looked over her Avon Collectibles. "They would make good gifts," he said, "if I just had someone to give them to." He glanced around the room and spotted an unoccupied table near the organ.

He walked over to the table and looked it over and then went back to visit with Emily again.

"Whose table is that over there?" he asked, as he pointed to Maria's table.

Bertha blurted it out before Emily could get her mouth open. "It's Maria's, and I don't know how she expects to make a sale when she's not even in here. She should have waited until it was over! She has no sense of salesmanship whatsoever."

"Sometimes a person just can't wait, Bertha." Sarah knew why Maria had dashed to her apartment, but did the whole Community Room and a Baptist pastor have to know?

Pastor Paul looked over Emily's Avon again more carefully and with sudden interest this time. He found an angel carrying a little harp, and Emily wrapped it in tissue paper, and he slipped it into his pocket. Just as he finished paying, Maria came back into the room.

"You had a customer while you were gone, Maria, but now he's spent his money elsewhere," Bertha announced in her loudest voice.

"Couldn't be helped. Is the buyer still here?" Maria asked anyone who was listening.

Just then Pastor Paul arrived at her table. "Yes, I'm still here, Maria, and I see you have a couple videos of the Gaithers. Are you really parting with them?"

Maria was instantly flustered. "Well, hello there. I missed you . . . oh, I mean, I guess I missed out on a sale, according to Bertha. But, yes, they are for sale." She recovered enough to sensibly ask, "Do you like the Gaithers, too?"

"Absolutely love them, and I don't have these particular ones. Oh, here's the one of Mark Lowry on Broadway. Isn't that a kick? And that Sandi Patty, what a voice! Are you sure you want to get rid of these?" He looked askance at her and frowned.

Maria assured him that she did, and he assured her that if she ever wanted to view them again, she could borrow them, or "We could watch them together," he whispered, as he leaned over to pay her and close the sale.

She was flustered again. "My eyes are getting bad," and that was all she could think of to say to discourage him. Yet, she wasn't sure if she really wanted to discourage him, and at her age, was it wise to play the old romantic game of "hard to get?" Maybe she could visit with him now and then. At least she still had her hearing.

Pastor Paul lingered for what seemed like an eternity. Finally, he said, "Well, I had better be going. I need to polish my sermon for tomorrow."

"Your sermon? I thought you were retired," Maria asked, as she closed her money box and began to clear off her table.

"Haven't you heard, Maria? Old preachers never retire; they're just put out to pasture." He laughed and smoothed his mustache. Maria's frown signaled her failure to get the joke. "It's a little play on words—pasture—pastor, get it?" He laughed again and rubbed his bald head. He continued, "I don't suppose you would want to go with me to church tomorrow. It's at the Little White Church on the Rogue. You know, just up I-5 a few miles."

Oh dear, how do I get out of this? Maria had hoped he wouldn't get around to that just yet. He really caught her off guard, and she had to come up with an excuse quickly, or she could accept and then get deathly sick by morning and cancel. Oh, what to do? Oh, what to do?

"In all honesty, Pastor Paul, I just don't think I can go tomorrow. You see, I am having company, and I am not just sure what time they are arriving. So, I thank you for the invitation, but will just have to beg off this time." Whew! Quick thinking, old girl, she thought.

Well, it could be true. One never knows when someone will pop in, and she had been spending occasional Sundays with her son and family, and although it was usually at their house, they could change plans and come to her place. How quickly she rationalized it all out in her head!

"Right. Well, it is short notice. Short notice for me to get a sermon ready, too. I just got the call yesterday that their pastor had a kidney transplant. I could be there for quite a few Sundays, so maybe you would like to go another time."

"We'll talk about it, okay?" Maria hoped she wasn't being too bold to suggest that, but it put him off for now. "My daughter is coming next month for a visit, so I will be busy, too."

He wanted to ask about her daughter and their religious views, and he had a million more questions, but it was not the time nor the place, and so he said good-bye. The other ladies were nearly packed up and ready to leave for their apartments.

Except for Millie. She was gushing with excitement. "Now we can have the boutique!"

CHAPTER NINETEEN

The Cat Comes Back

"April prepares her green traffic light,
And the world thinks GO!"
—Christopher Marley

Her withered lips kissed the bathroom mirror. Cat's coming! Cat's coming! For the first time in weeks, Maria felt truly happy. She'd been treading water since nearly drowning in the deluge when Cat left in February, but she had managed to keep her head above water and her eye on the lighthouse of the distant days until Cat's return. It would always be this way. Cat's coming and going and happiness and sadness. Unless, of course, she and Tony made something of their lives together. Maybe Cat would move to Middleford, but Maria had no clue really as to how their relationship was going. She saw Tony around the facility, but he was always in a hurry to fix something or clean a floor, so Maria stayed out of his way.

Cat was fairly tight-lipped about their relationship, although at first she told Maria they communicated every day. Maria had never been a prying mother, and she wasn't going to start now. Cat would tell her as much as she thought she needed to know when she wanted her to know. As close as they were, they respected each other's privacy, and Maria admired her daughter for that.

When Cat arrived in the afternoon on Thursday, April 5, Maria was the one who greeted her out front. Cat had called Maria on her cell phone and said she'd be there in 30 minutes, so Maria bustled out to the bench and waited. She saw a flash of red and heard the familiar honking of the horn, and for the first time in weeks, Maria glowed like the bright orb of sunshine that was pulsing down and heating the April flowers that Tony had planted amongst the shrubbery all around the building. Spring had been worth waiting for, after all.

Maria couldn't wait for Cat to get settled in, so they could sit and talk and drink the mochas that Cat had bought on her way into town. She wanted to tell her in detail all that had been happening in the last few weeks, and she was equally anxious to catch up on Cat's life. But first they had to politely smile and greet those in the lobby who were awaiting Cat's return as well.

Millie was just arriving home from a shopping trip and heard the commotion and saw a cluster of ladies. "What did you say, Sarah? Something about a cat being back? Who around here has a cat? I . . ." Just then she spotted Maria and her daughter. "Oh, hello, dear. Oh, yes, your name is Cat, isn't it? Well, welcome home!" Millie gushed and kissed Cat on the cheek. "Oh, say, did I ever tell you about the audition I had for a part in *Cat on a Hot Tin Roof?* I was . . ."

Maria interrupted her and excused them both as politely as she could by saying that Cat had driven for hours and needed to rest, and off they went, each dragging a suitcase to Maria's apartment.

After tending to necessary business, they settled in on the couch with mochas in hand and began to talk. Maria skipped the part about her depression and launched into a lengthy story of Pastor Paul's advances, the Spring Cleaning Sale, and Millie's boutique. "She had it all set up and ready to open on Sunday after the sale, but then when Sherrie came in on Monday, she told her she couldn't do it. She couldn't have a boutique at all! You should have seen Millie pouting and Bertha gloating."

Cat figured Bertha had put the kibosh on it, but Maria said, "No, it had something to do with the rules and regulations made by the government. Millie threatened to move out, but we all talked her into staying. She drives us nuts, but she is quite an interesting character. Oh, I haven't talked this much in weeks, Cat. You have no idea how glad I am that you're here." She reached over and grabbed Cat's hand.

"Me too," Cat yawned. "I missed you a lot, Mom," and she squeezed Maria's hand in return. "I mean, I really missed you."

"And Tony," Maria added.

"Ah, yes, Tony," Cat said with hesitation. We e-mailed and talked on the phone, but I just don't know about him. I came back now because I told him I would come for Pear Blossom weekend, but I have to test the waters. I'm not too sure about him. He could be boring, but we'll see. I'll call him later. He had to go to Grants Pass for a meeting today."

Cat was anxious to change the subject. "So tell me more about Pastor Paul."

They had a couple quick dinners that Maria proudly microwaved. "See, I learned how to cook in it," she told Cat, and then they talked long into the evening about everything, and Maria felt relaxed and happy once again. Cat even forgot about calling Tony.

"I have a surprise for you, Mom, but I'll tell you about it first thing tomorrow, okay?"

"What a thing to say and right at bedtime! Now, I'll be wound up all night and won't sleep a wink. Come on; at least give me a little hint." That was typical of Cat.

Cat couldn't think of anything that wouldn't give it away. "Patience, little one. That's what you used to tell me. Now, go to bed, and I'll tell you manana."

Maria was curious and exasperated, "Oh well, at least I know you're not pregnant! Are you?"

*   *   *

Maria awoke refreshed for the first time in weeks. She smiled as she sat on the edge of the bed and stretched, daring her arthritis to constrain the energy she felt. She forgot her age and tried to hop up and run into the living room, but the muscles in her legs screamed, "I'm still here, old girl. Slow down!" She heard the phone ring and bent over to answer it.

"Hi, it's me. Tony. I thought you were going to call me last night, Cat."

Maria hung up when she heard Cat answering him on the phone in the living room, and she supposed Cat's whole day would be taken up with him. Her mood changed quickly, and she plopped back down on the bed.

In just a few minutes, though, Cat knocked on the bedroom door and entered cautiously, thinking her mother might be cat-napping, but Maria motioned her over to sit on the bed.

"Good morning. Are you bright-eyed and bushy-tailed, Mom? I thought we could go out for breakfast." She kissed Maria on the forehead.

"Hi, there. Oh, I am so glad you are here, Cat. Did I tell you that?"

'Yeah, a couple times, but I like hearing it and I love being here. Now, come on and get up. I'm starving."

Although Maria didn't like to hurry around in the mornings, she loved to go out for breakfast, and within one hour they were both ready to go out the door.

"But what about Tony? I thought you would be spending all day with him."

"Nope. It's Friday. Still a work day for him, and he has to run down to Ashland this morning, so I haven't even seen him yet." Maria thought Cat sounded almost relieved.

"He gets off at 4:00, so then we are going for a drive. I have to see him sooner or later, I guess, before we leave."

"*We leave?*"

"Yes, that's the surprise; Come on. I'll tell you over the bacon and eggs."

Archie's Diner was across town, and Cat hurriedly sped through one yellow light after another. She was used to driving that way and never got stopped.

Maria was horrified at her driving. "You know, they have cameras now, and they can record everything and send you a ticket right through the mail. I know because it happened to Jillian."

Cat just laughed and said, "I'm just too fast for the shutter to click."

"Well, don't blame me if you get a ticket in the mail. I warned you."

The diner was thinning out after the early morning rush, and Cat and Maria were shown to a small table by the window. Neither one of them had been there before, but Maria had heard from Millie that they served good breakfasts and were reasonably priced.

"Actually, Millie used the word *cheap*. I think that just . . . well, cheapens the whole idea of it. But then she likes to eat at the truck stop and see the men. She says if you have a certain demeanor about you, they will never bother you. Just visit with them, but act in control at all times."

"So, does she practice that demeanor?" Cat asked. Just from the little bit she had seen and heard of Millie, she figured Millie could act any part she wanted.

Maria was tired of that conversation. "I don't know, Cat, and I really don't care. Now, let's order and then tell me the surprise." When she was through with a subject, it abruptly ended.

So, over hash browns, bacon crisply fried, and scrambled eggs, Cat told Maria that she had a free-lance writing job on the Oregon Coast, and she wanted Maria to go with her. "I thought we could leave on Sunday, drive over to Florence and stay there that night, and then work on Monday there, go on down the coast as far as Bandon, and work on the way. We'd probably come back on Wednesday. So, what do you think, Mom? Want to be my apprentice?"

"Oh, my gosh. How exciting! Of course, I'll go," Maria hadn't been this excited since Jillian had her baby girl. "What do you mean we'll work? I don't know how to write." And then her worries kicked in. "But it's so sudden, and we'd be leaving so soon. I would have so much to do to get ready. Oh no. I couldn't possible go." Marie's excitement turned to fears and defeat. "And it would cost so much. Oh no! It's not in my budget. I'll have to stay home, Cat."

"Now, what in the world is keeping you home?" Cat was used to her mother backing out, but this was utterly ridiculous. She hadn't even told her that the next assignment was in Italy, and she would pay her way, if she'd go with her there, too. She'd spring that on her later.

Finally over their third cups of coffee, Cat convinced her mother to travel with her to the coast. "We'll wash clothes, and I'll help you pack, and the trip won't cost you a dime. Since the assignment is to write about quaint little restaurants on the way, our meals are free, and we'll have twin beds at the magazine's expense."

"There's only one problem with all those plans, Cat." Maria was laughing, as she pointed out to Cat that *she* would wash the clothes after the fiasco with the quarters last time Cat tried to do the laundry. "That poor woman still talks about how that machine went on and on."

*   *   *

Cat and Tony picked up their race packets and attended the pasta feed on Friday, and they spent most of Saturday together at the Pear Blossom Festival. They ran in the two mile race, enjoyed the parade, and walked through the Street Faire. Maria was far too busy to take in any of it, and since Josie's float idea had fallen through due to insurance problems, very few of the residents participated in it either. Oscar had a watercolor "hanging," at the theater, Antonio entered the chili cook-off, and Sarah helped with the book sale at the public library. Other than that, most residents stayed around "the home."

Pastor Paul showed up in the laundry room right when Maria was folding her freshly washed unmentionables. She quickly tossed them in her laundry basket and covered them with a clean bath towel. Now her undies would be wrinkled, which right there was something practically against her religion! His timing was very poor. He asked her again to attend church with him, but her daughter won out over his advances. "Well, maybe next time," he said for the second time. "I'll be there preaching for at least two months." He wasn't going to give up on Maria. Her excuses seemed perfectly logical and acceptable so far, and the Lord had taught him perseverance in all things, so he would steadfastly pursue her. He couched his thoughts in biblical terms. Since the Lord had shown him how to never give up and to run the race with a goal in mind, it sounded so much better to think in those ways than to say he was chasing an old broad! Oh yes, when she got home from the coast, there would be a surprise hanging on her doorknob.

*   *   *

And so, while Maria and Cat were enjoying the trip to and from the coast—the scenery, the food, and each other's company—life went on at Pear Blossom. Essie prowled around all hours of the night, Winnie burned her beans and wondered where all the smoke was coming from, and the Bird Woman sat by the hour and fondled her coin collection. She still wondered if somehow she should bury it in a coffee can. Oscar had another spell and took a ride in the ambulance, Sarah's acute allergy attack sent her off to her doctor for a shot, and Gayle's dog had another accident in the lobby. Pastor Paul was busy designing a card and choosing poetry.

CHAPTER TWENTY

Josie's Disappointment

"Seated one day at the organ,
I was weary and ill at ease,
And my fingers wandered idly
Over the noisy keys."
—Adelaide Ann Proctor

Josie was tasting her first mouthful of defeat with her senior project, and it left a bitter, caustic aftertaste that hovered for hours and even days. No amount of toothpaste or mouthwash could ever be strong enough to remove the residue, and no amount of head-shaking and disbelief could erase the nasty words that stuck like velcro in Josie's head.

She had spent an afternoon with Bertha. Only the Lord could help Josie understand that woman and forgive her.

Sherrie had a list of things that Josie could begin working on—redoing the boring bulletin board with timely, colorful borders and pictures; cleaning the library shelves and organizing the books; helping residents plant their flower boxes; and helping Betty plan the next major activity for the month of May, the dog birthday party. The last item on the list was to help residents clean their apartments, and when Josie saw Bertha's name at the top of the list, she knew what her first part of her project would be. Sherrie tried to talk her out of it and steer her into something easier than having to deal with Bertha's attitudes and opinions right away. Maybe she could work into that later, but Josie was convinced in her mind and adamant in her words to Sherrie that Bertha was her first choice. How could she figure Bertha out and try to help her like herself if she was lining up construction paper on a bulletin board or rearranging the Harlequin Romance novels in the library?

"No, I want to jump right in and help Bertha. I'll get to know her by visiting while cleaning her kitchen cupboards, washing her linens, or whatever else in Bertha's apartment needs attention," Josie told Sherrie, eagerly.

For starters, Bertha was none too happy when she found out that Josie would be helping her, and when Josie arrived for her duties, Bertha looked up and down the hallway before she let her in. "You didn't bring that Mongoloid, did you?" She growled at Josie.

"No, my little brother is home playing baseball with his daddy right now, and it is called Down Syndrome, not Mongoloid." Josie felt she had already started off all wrong. She had been taught not to correct her elders, but also she had been taught to stick up for her brother and those like him. "He's really a sweet little boy, and you know, he can't help the way he is."

There was no persuading Bertha that Jake had a valuable place in society. "He should be put away somewhere. I suppose the next thing I'll hear is that he goes to school."

Josie was happy to report that, "Yes, he goes to the same Christian school that I go to. There is a special education class there for him, and he loves it. He has learned so much!" Josie said proudly. "Last week he learned how to tie his shoes," Josie beamed with delight.

Bertha was relieved to hear, at least, that his parents were paying at a private school for him to tie his shoes, and her tax dollars weren't going to help him learn something that could be taught at home. "How ridiculous!" she expounded. "What will ever become of him? He'll just be a burden on society." But Josie assured her that he would never be institutionalized or on welfare; she herself would dedicate her whole life to him, if that's what it took.

The afternoon wore on, and somewhere amongst the cleaning of the cinnamon and nutmeg containers, and the jars of parsley and oregano, and the flour and sugar canisters in Bertha's kitchen, even more of Bertha's venom spewed forth, and this time she attacked her fellow residents and Sherrie, the administrator. She had nothing nice to say about any of them. In fact, she tore each one to shreds like cat claws sliding down a sheer curtain. Few in the facility were spared her diatribe and ridicule until finally Josie had heard enough.

Politely, she glanced at her watch, and thankfully it was dinner time at home, so she had a good reason to leave. Josie felt as bruised as the Bird Woman had after a beating from her grandson, but the black and blue marks were for others, for those who had to live near Bertha and listen to her, day after sickening day. She felt sick to her stomach as she drove home to her safe haven and loving family's arms. She prayed as she drove across town and what struck her as she pulled into the driveway at home was how God kept turning her prayers into supplications and help for Bertha, not for those around her.

Maybe someday she'd ask God again to help her with Bertha, but right then she wasn't up to another day with that woman! I'll pray for her, but that's all for right now, Josie thought, as she ran up the front steps and massaged her aching forehead. Not only does Bertha not like herself, she doesn't like *anybody* else! The question remained, "But why not?"

Josie was not over her aching heart at the sing-a-long on Wednesday night. As much as she still wanted Bertha to get help for her self-image, she really hoped deep down that Bertha would find something else to do that evening. She just wasn't ready to see or hear her again just yet.

Josie arrived early to practice a few numbers, and her frustration and upset feelings came out as she banged out the notes like a rag-time piano player.

"What is that horrible noise?" She heard a distinctive voice and saw the glint of the wheelchair's metal, and she knew the fun(?) had begun. "You didn't bring that Mongoloid, did you?" Bertha scanned the room quickly. Noticing Josie's frowning face and shaking head, Bertha discovered her mistake herself. "Down Syndrome, Up Syndrome. What does it matter? Everything is called a *syndrome* these days. At least my ailment had a name for itself—polio!"

"Polio? You had polio?" Josie's fingers came up off the keyboard like she had been shot in the arms. "Oh, I'm sorry, Bertha. I had no idea you had polio!"

"No reason to be sorry. It's not your fault. I've lived with the residue of it for70 years, and I never complain!"

No, not about that; just about everything and everyone else, Josie thought. So, was that what had hardened Bertha's heart? Was this little crack the chink in her armor that Josie could pry apart and get to Bertha's soul? Actually, it was a big admission on Bertha's part. Not many people at Pear Blossom knew about Bertha's past or just why she was wheelchair bound. They were too afraid to ask, and she had made it perfectly clear that if she wanted people to know about her, she would tell them. She firmly believed in the "don't ask, don't tell" policy.

Other residents were starting to filter in, so Bertha wheeled away to her usual spot, and Josie settled in at the keyboard. She relaxed when she saw the friendly faces of Essie and Sarah, and she gave a great big smile to Maria and Cat who had just barely made it back from the coast in time. Winnie stomped in right on the dot, but Millie had suffered the effects of her hot prune juice cocktail all day, so she was late and a little nervous to be there at all. Others came and went and clapped and sang, and the evening turned out to be fun for all involved—even Josie.

The evening wound down, and Josie played *Danny Boy* as a final request for Sarah. Essie was crying, and the Bird Woman was sorting through the table of freebies hoping to find a coffee can. But it was Bertha who lingered the longest for a final word with Josie.

"Wait a minute, would you? Come here," and Bertha pulled Josie low over her chair, so she could whisper in her ear. "Don't tell anyone about my condition, the P word. It just slipped out, and nobody needs to know." Bertha was almost pleading with a slight softness to her voice that Josie had not heard before.

Josie assured her that it was their little secret, and she went out the door with hope in her heart that the next time she tried to help Bertha, God would put words in Josie's mouth to begin to heal the aches from which Bertha must have been hurting all those years. Tenderness, forgiveness, grace, hope, joy, and most of all love—Josie herself was just beginning to understand God's goodness and His teachings in all these areas, and now she wanted so desperately to share them with Bertha.

"In *my* time, little one. In *my* time." God had to pull on the reins to hold Josie back.

CHAPTER TWENTY-ONE

Windows of Opportunity

"A woman's time of opportunity is short,
And if she doesn't seize it, no one wants to
Marry her, and she sits watching for omens."
—Aristophanes

"Italy? We just got back from the coast, and now you spring a trip to Italy on me. Cat, you never cease to amaze me—but no, I can't go. That is too far away!" Maria hadn't even unpacked her toothbrush. "And I'm too tired," she added.

"Plus, now you have a sweetie who leaves angels on your doorknob." Cat was ready for all her mother's negative answers for the proposed trip to Italy in the fall. Might as well tell her now, so she'll have plenty of time to worry, Cat had decided.

Maria ignored Cat's comment about the angels on the doorknob and went blithely on her way arranging her cosmetics in the bathroom vanity and storing her unused nightgowns in the dresser drawer.

Zipping her suitcase shut, she said with resignation, "There, that's done until my next trip, and Lord knows when that will be with you gallivanting off to other countries. By the way, what about your sweetie? How can you leave Tony?"

Cat knew this was coming. "Oh, that won't be too hard since I'm not around much anyway." She hoped that answer would satisfy her mother for the time being, but in all reality, she had decided that Tony would be a friend and that would be all. She was rather enjoying her life as a single woman. Her writing had become her passion and her focus, and she didn't need a man distracting her. They really had nothing in common except Pear Blossom, but even with that, his intrigue with the heating system of the facility and the sprinkler system did nothing to flip-flop her heart. The word that fit him was *boring*, and although it was not the most eloquent word for a writer to use, it summed up his qualities. A nice man, but boring.

"Seems like you are playing hard-to-get." Maria was not done with Cat and Tony just yet. "I've always heard that's the best way to snag a man, although I could never understand the logic in that. Seems like it would drive them off, but I suppose those egos need a big challenge."

"Touche! Seems like that is the way you are playing with Pastor Paul, but it might not be good for you, Mom. The window of opportunity might close, never to be opened again."

"Sure, because I am so old. Is that what you are saying? Okay, yes, he is pursuing me, I guess you could say, and yes, it is kind of fun. I admit it, but it is also scary. A woman of my age! What if I get attached to him, and he gets sick or even worse, what if he dies? Oh, shoot! I don't even know him. All I know is that he's a Baptist, and I'm a Presbyterian, and those two would never work! And there's no changing me at this age!"

"Did you read the card that came with this little angel figurine, Mom? He really sounds serious."

Maria shrugged, sat down hard on the couch, and turned her face toward Cat. "No, read away, dear. What did the old boy write this time?"

"This he quotes from someone named Jerome," and Cat began to read.

"'Nothing, so it seems to me,' said the stranger, 'is more beautiful than the love that has weathered the storms of life . . . The love of the young for the young, that is the beginning of life. But the love of the old for the old, that is the beginning of—of things longer.' Maria, will you weather the storms with me? With love, Pastor Paul"

"Mom, I think he just proposed to you!" Cat's face registered surprise and pleasure.

"Nonsense! Don't take everything so literally, Cat. Maybe he just wants to sit outside on the bench with me in different kinds of weather! You know, feel the sun, smell the rain . . . that sort of thing." She tried to sound convincing for Cat's sake, but she didn't sound believable even to herself.

"I would say the window of opportunity has been thrown wide open for you, Mom, and you'd better let the sunshine in." Cat was excited and showed it, while Maria tried to calm the school-girl butterflies that threatened to fly in all directions at once. "Let me see your neck." Cat approached her mother and pulled open the neckline of her mother's blouse. "Yep, it's red like a flashing light. That's always been a dead giveaway of your nervous reactions, Mom."

"Nonsense! It's just the red dye rubbing off of this new blouse. I knew that cheap store on the coast sold inferior goods. I just wasted my money." Maria's attempts at covering up Cat's knowledge and feelings of what was really true was about as good as a tornado covering up its destructive path.

"Okay, be in denial, Mom, if you want. It's lonely there. I lived there for several years when I was married. Denying the obvious facts of infidelity, drugs, and booze of my husband, which, of course, were much bigger things and more destructive to deny than your little romance with the pastor. All I'm saying is, Mom, that I don't want you to be lonely, and here is a seemingly nice man who wants to spend time with you. So I hope you will at least give him a chance. Go to church with him, cook dinner for him, get to know him." Cat was being the mother now.

"Oh, my gosh, Cat. I've been playing so hard to get that I haven't even thanked him for the Valentine or the poetry or the flowers. There, I admitted it. But what must he think of me and my lack of manners?"

"I'd say by his persistence that all is forgiven. Oh, I just had a brilliant idea! Find out what time he's preaching on Sunday, and we'll go to church and check out his sermons."

Maria needed time to think that one over, but it would be an ice-breaker, and she'd feel more comfortable sitting in a pew with Cat than showing up on his arm and waiting by herself while he attended to his pastoral duties.

The next morning while Cat was still asleep, Maria adjusted her magnifying glass just right and scanned the Yellow Pages of the Rogue Valley phone book. After much squinting and determination, she dialed the secretarial office of the little white church up I-5 that Pastor Paul had described. A deep, male voice answered the phone. "The Little White Church on the Rogue. Pastor Paul here. What can I help you with today?"

Maria stuttered and stammered and tried to change her voice to make it sound younger.

"Ma'am, is something wrong? Do you need help?" Pastor Paul didn't recognize the high-pitched, whiney voice nor could he figure out what the caller wanted.

"What time is church on Sunday?" Maria finally blurted out her request, so it was understandable. She would never have called if she'd known he was the interim secretary, too.

"Is this Maria?" Pastor Paul noted a tone of voice that he was beginning to recognize and longing to hear.

"Well, yes, I guess it is," she said and gave a nervous, little laugh at the same time. "I'm sorry to bother you. I was looking for the secretary."

"Oh, Maria, go right ahead and bother me." Oh, how you bother my heart, he was thinking. "Do you need me for something?" How I hope so! His thoughts were begging.

"Well, my daughter is here visiting, and she was just wondering what time church services are on Sunday. She thought we might attend. You know, just to see . . ."

"Bless her heart for thinking that way. Yes, do come! We start around 10:30 with coffee and visiting, and then the worship service is at 11:00. Of course, now, if you'd like to come for Sunday School too, that's at 9:30. We have an adult class, and we're studying . . ."

Maria hated to interrupt him, but really a church service would be enough of a start. "We'll just come for church, thank you," she said too abruptly. Her embarrassment caused her to speak in harsh tones and short statements so she could get off the phone.

"See you then, if not before," she added. "Oh, and thank you for the angel figurine and the card." Suddenly, she remembered her manners, and now the phone call had become something more than a business call to seek information. "I have been going to write you a note for all your niceties toward me, but I have been lax. I really do appreciate all your gifts. I hope you will forgive me."

"Ah, forgiveness. That is the subject we are studying in Sunday School. You would be an A student if you came. So, yes, of course, I forgive you. No need to write a note, Maria. I just hope you liked the flowers and the poetry, too."

"I have loved it all, but, of course, for quite some time, I had no idea that the little gifts were from you. When I found out, I was quite astonished." Maria was babbling along like Bear Creek that wound its way through Middleford. Her flowing chatter hadn't quite reached the proportions of the rambling Rogue River, but if she didn't shut it off soon, she would inundate the poor man with her words.

"It's good to hear all this, Maria." Pastor Paul did not share in her fears of prattling on. It was music to his ears. "And just who did you think was leaving gifts for you?"

"Antonio . . . Oh, I mean Tony. You know Tony, the maintenance man. He took a shine to my daughter Cat right away, and we . . . well, I thought they were from Tony for Cat, and then to complicate matters, some *were* from him. Anyway, now it is all straightened out, and I thank you again." Maria was even more anxious to end this conversation because Cat was standing in front of her with her face in contortions trying to figure out who was on the other end of the phone cord and why her mother was telling that person about Tony's infatuation with her.

"See you Sunday morning, then," and with that Maria hung up.

"Well, that's all out in the open now, and I do feel relieved." Maria brushed her hand across her forehead. "And we're going to church on Sunday! Oh dear, what about my hair and my nails? Do you think I can get any appointments this late in the week? Oh, Cat, what have I done? Here it is Thursday, and I only have three days to get ready. What will I wear?"

Cat was still rubbing the sleep from her eyes. "Sounds to me like you've taken control like you used to do. I can kink your hair and polish your nails, you know."

"Cat, you know I would call on you in a minute to do them, but for this I really need a professional. You see, dear, I haven't been to church in years. I wish ladies still wore hats. That would solve the hair problem."

"The young gals wear baseball caps with the ponytail sticking out in the back," Cat informed her mother of the latest style.

"Jillian does that, but not at church! Oh, heavens no! Just what church have you been attending, Cat, to see something like that?"

"Haven't been lately . . . skipped a couple Sundays . . . slept in . . . had to work . . ."

"Okay. That's enough excuses. I can't criticize because I've been delinquent, too. No car . . . no friends to take me . . . poor eyesight to read the Bible . . . can't sing . . . Don't we sound like poor, pitiful Pearl with all our excuses, Cat? Oh, cry me a river."

"The Rogue River, of course!" Cat added.

CHAPTER TWENTY-TWO

Maria's Rebirth

"Just when the caterpillar
thought the world was over,
it became a butterfly."
—Anonymous

Life was slowly plodding along in the mundane world of most of the residents at Pear Blossom. Drink the coffee, read the paper, take the pills, make another doctor's appointment, gripe to the neighbors, check the mail, microwave a meal, walk up and down the halls if able, and then fall into bed and hope to wake up the next morning, and do it all over again.

Winnie loved her liquor, Gayle walked her dog, and the Bird Woman polished her coins and kept looking for empty coffee cans. Millie unearthed her swimsuits, so she'd be ready for old sol to tan her sagging skin, and Betty rearranged the bulletin board. Sarah's acid reflux was keeping her awake nights, and Emily busily ordered more Avon products.

Oscar and Otis had retreated into their shells again, and Antonio spent time admiring his latest trophy from the chili contest. Essie was waiting for Josie Winters to come and clean her apartment, and Bertha was overseeing the whole facility and all the other residents and reporting to Sherrie.

But nobody was as busy as Maria. With appointments made for Friday morning with a new hairdresser and nail technician and with a pedicurist in the afternoon, all Maria had to worry about was her wardrobe. Cat didn't care what she herself would wear. All she brought, and all she ever wore were sports clothes, so the Baptists would just have to put up with her black Adidas warm-up jacket and jogging pants. Maria rolled her eyes and shook her head.

She hoped when they went out shopping that Cat might accidentally run across something a little more feminine and dressy. I'll pay for it if I have to, Maria resigned herself to the fact that if she wanted Cat to look presentable on Sunday, she would have to take control.

"What do you wear when you meet with your publishers? You must dress up for business engagements, don't you?" Maria hoped she had instilled some sense of pride and decorum in her daughter's choice of clothing, but Cat had never worried much about styles and colors. She liked to be comfortable and casual, and most of her work she did at home on the computer.

"Don't worry, Mom. I must look okay. They wouldn't hire me on my writing alone. I do have a dark jacket with matching slacks, and it even has a skirt, although I've never worn it. I wear a white blouse and dress it up with that red scarf you gave me."

"None of which you brought, I suppose. And what about shoes? You can't go clunking into Pastor Paul's church in those tennis shoes!" Maria was getting more horrified by the moment with Cat's lack of style and her diminished wardrobe. "I'll be mortified!"

Maria loved to look through the ads in the Sunday paper and check out the colors and the seasonal wardrobe offerings for women. When she watched the beauty pageants on television, she was more enamored with what the gals wore than with their beauty or their talent. Her dreams of being a model were dashed when she had suddenly stopped growing taller in the eighth grade, but nevertheless, she had always been a stylish woman.

*   *   *

The Middleford Mall was fairly quiet that Thursday afternoon as Maria and Cat perused the women's clothing sections of the major department stores and found very little that appealed to either of them. Maria needed the Full-Figured departments, while Cat leaned toward the sportswear sections, and Maria had to pull her back.

Finally, after a light lunch at the food court, Maria suggested they check out her favorite clothing store on the second floor—Carlotta's, and it was there under the watchful eye of Carlotta herself and Maria, as her understudy, that Cat found a long, flowered, full skirt with a matching top. The shades of red looked stunning with her dark hair. Cat twirled like little Shirley Temple had done in her movies, but it was just a good show for her mother. At least the fullness of the skirt and the elastic waistband were comfortable.

Maria found a long skirt, too, with pastel colors, and she was quite sure she had a blouse at home to match. With having to buy Cat's outfit, she would forego getting a new top, but Cat had seen her mother looking longingly at the matching knit shell, and being quicker than Maria, had her credit card swiped through the machine for all the purchases before Maria could find her checkbook. Maria argued vehemently, but it was too late.

"What about shoes? That is still a problem. Do you think you could squish your toes into some of mine, Cat?"

"Actually, I did bring some white loafers. They would work, huh?"

"What? Wear white before Memorial Day? Have all the rules changed?" Maria was mortified. "And what about a handbag? It has to match the shoes, you know." Maria had a kaleidoscope of matching footwear and purses.

"How about if I just toss my car keys and driver's license in your purse when we get there? I really don't need a bag, do I?"

"I give up. If you want to be underdressed and incomplete, I guess I shouldn't worry. After all, Pastor Paul will be looking at me."

"Oh, yes, and be sure to wear your earrings, Mother. We don't want you to be naked!"

The beauty appointments on Friday consumed the day, and Maria was exhausted when they returned to Pear Blossom. Cat and Tony were going out to dinner at Red Lobster, and Cat wanted her mother to come with them, but Maria was too tired. "No, I must save myself for Sunday, and besides you don't need an old woman to tag along on a date. I'll just get rested up so I don't sleep through church. Wouldn't that be awful if I snored? Oh, Cat, don't let me snore. Jab me in the ribs or something. Will you promise to do that?"

Cat laughed. "The things you worry about, Mom. I think you will be too excited to sleep through Pastor Paul's sermon. Now, try to relax while I'm gone tonight. Play cards with the girls or take a nap."

"I'll pass on the card games this week. What if I would grab for a card and break a nail?"

And so Maria had an evening of catnaps, mixed in with a Daniel O'Donnell special on PBS and a bowl of popcorn. What if I break a tooth? she thought, but decided to live dangerously.

*　　*　　*

The next morning when Maria and Cat entered the Community Room with a bowl of grapes for the Saturday morning Koffee Klatch, Sarah and

Betty were the only ones present. They wondered why Maria hadn't joined them for UNO the night before.

When Sarah found out that *Danny*, as she called him with unabashed love and familiarity, had been on PBS, she became very upset. "I wonder why I didn't know that. You know, I am a charter member of his fan club. I even went to his wedding! Well, actually, I watched a video of it, but I felt like I was right there, and have you ever heard him sing to his mother? She is quite elderly, you know, and he is so good to her. Maybe that's why I like him so well." She could have gone on for hours about the merits of his voice and the benefits of belonging to his fan club, but then Millie arrived, and she heard the word *club*. She had one white hearing aide in, for a change.

"Well, I belong to Harry and David's Fruit of the Month Club. They send fruit every Christmas for me to all my friends in California. Oh, speaking of California, last week a couple came up from L.A. and took me to dinner on Saturday night. It was nice, but I missed the Lawrence Welk show." Millie's lower lip protruded into a pout that the Bird Woman could have perched on.

By now, Bertha had arrived. "You just pout to get attention, but you're not funny, Millie. Anyone can belong to the Fruit of the Month Club. It's not as exclusive as you make it sound, and you've seen all those Lawrence Welk shows over and over. They're just repeats."

Millie stuck up for what she liked, and not even Bertha could dissuade her love for the songs of that era, the fancy dresses, and beautiful stage settings. "Well, I'll have you know, Miss Know-It-All, that I've sung some of those songs myself, worn the ball gowns and been on more stages than you could ever imagine, so if I want to watch it, it's none of your business!"

Maria was getting distraught over Millie and Bertha's tirades. "Cat, maybe we should leave. I don't want to get too nervous and perspire and have all the curl come out of my hair."

But before they could get up out of their chairs, Betty joined in. "Oh, this is nothing. You should have been here last night. Essie and Winnie really got into it."

Maria's interest was piqued, and she settled back to hear Betty's story. "Okay. What did I miss? Or do I really want to know? I hope I won't get too upset."

Betty was determined to tell the story even though most of them had heard it, ad nauseam.

"To start from the beginning, last fall Winnie got angry with Essie over the way she works the puzzles." Betty waved her hand over in the direction of the big, oak table where a 1,000 piece puzzle of the Sistine Chapel was under construction. "Poor Essie drops the pieces on the floor or leans over, and they stick to her clothes. Anyway, Winnie didn't like it and told Essie, so they had a big fight. Essie started doing a puzzle the next day on another table, and Winnie had a fit and went to Sherrie about it. Sherrie told her we can use as many tables as we want. Winnie had never used that table. She never even liked that table. So Winnie decided that Essie was mentally unbalanced and refused to do anything with Essie. She wouldn't even play cards if Essie was going to play. So up until last night, Winnie had started her own card games with others of her ilk, and our card games have been rather nice without Winnie changing the rules to suit herself, wouldn't you agree, girls?" They all nodded in agreement, except for Winnie's bosom buddy, Bertha. She glared at Betty, daring her to go on.

Betty stopped for breath and to gather her wits about her for the crux of the story of last night. "Who should show up and want to play cards with us, but Winnie. Her group was all busy with other things. Well, there sat poor Essie, looking all bewildered and scared. We began the game, and guess what happened? Essie dropped her cards on the floor, and Winnie began to scream. She finally settled down, but then when Essie played a Draw Four card, and Winnie was on her last two cards and then had to draw four, she fell apart at the seams. You mean, Maria, that you didn't hear Winnie shouting? She stuck her tongue out at Essie and then got up and left the room and was yelling all the way down past your door."

Maria said, "I must have been having a nice nap and snoring so loudly that I didn't hear anything. I'm so glad I missed it; Winnie sounds like she's the one mentally unbalanced!"

Cat was busy scribbling notes on a small notepad she had pulled from her pocket. "More fodder for my book," she whispered in her mother's ear. "Mixed nuts!"

The rest of Saturday was a calm day in the facility, although not so with Maria's nerves. She tried to keep busy, and she did a load of laundry *without* Cat's assistance, they went out for a mocha in the early afternoon, and Cat fixed a huge, green salad with garlic bread for dinner. Maria refused to eat the garlic bread. "What if it didn't get all out of my system overnight, and the odor would come out through my pores while we're singing *Amazing Grace* at church?"

"I thought you don't like to sing." Cat was laughing and crying at the same time.

"Well, I like to, but I just can't hit those notes. I will try to make a joyful noise for Pastor Paul's sake. 'I once was lost, but now am found. Was blind, but now I see.' I wish I *could* see better. Maybe I'd go to church every Sunday."

"I have a hunch you'll be a frequent visitor now, Mom. Tomorrow will tell the tale!"

*   *   *

With the same careful attention that Maria had taken with the preparations of her clothes, hair, and make-up, Pastor Paul had devoted extra hours to the cleanliness of the church and the preparation of the service. Although the church did have a paid janitor, Pastor Paul polished the pews with furniture wax, personally inspected the bathroom, and swept the front sidewalk—all on Sunday morning. He had printed up special, large-print bulletins, enlarged the words of each song that flashed on the screen up front, and made sure the hand-held listening devices were in good working order in case any of the parishioners were hard-of-hearing. He knew of Maria's eyesight problems, but was not sure of her hearing abilities. He didn't want her to miss a thing, although if he had known her very well at all, her pride would never let her admit a hearing loss by holding one of those receptors in her hand while he preached.

All was in order, Sunday School was over, and the pews were beginning to fill with the regulars. Pastor Paul was in the study upstairs, adjusting his tie for the hundredth time that morning and looking over his sermon notes. He could hear the organist playing softly and the buzzing voices of folks as they poured a cup of coffee and visited for a few moments before the worship service started. He wondered if Maria and Cat were there yet, but he had decided to wait and pick them out of the congregation when he got up in front. On a good Sunday there might be 75-80 in the sanctuary, and with it being close to Easter, the pews might possibly be full. "Forgive me, Lord," he prayed. "I will only have eyes for a couple people, well, actually, only one." Pastor Paul glanced at the clock. "Okay, Lord, let's have church!"

Maria and Cat tried not to be too early, but it was hard for Maria to get anywhere right on time. She knew she didn't want a cup of coffee to get her bladder all stimulated and over-active, so they by-passed the coffee pot and went right on into the sanctuary. They found two seats at the end of a pew, and as they sat down, Cat noticed someone waving from the other end of the row. It was Josie and Jake Winters. Jake was pointing at Cat, and Josie had to grab and hold his hands to keep him from clapping. Cat assumed the couple sitting by the kids must be the parents. Josie was just a younger version of the lady seated next to her.

"Who is it, dear? I didn't think we would know anyone here." Maria tried to crane her neck past Cat, but the eyestrain was just too hard on her.

"It's Josie and Jake and their parents, I guess. The kids seem glad to see us. Pretend you can see them and wave back." Maria did as she was told because she wanted to be friendly—and especially with those dear kids. "We'll visit with them afterwards," Cat assured her mother

Then the music swelled to a final note, and Pastor Paul stepped to the podium. Although Maria couldn't see the fine details of his face, she could hear his booming voice. It was smooth and melodious, yet strong and just loud enough for her ears. She sat back and relaxed as he welcomed the congregation, made announcements, and opened with a nice prayer. Maria could tell that it was from his heart and not just one he read from a script. The service went on with hymns, Scripture reading, a soloist, and another prayer, and then he began his sermon. She stayed awake easily and listened to every word. His rhythmic intonations seemed to bounce off the colors of the stained-glass windows and fill the room with sounds that filled her heart with joy. He was talking about being born again. Was she dreaming? No, she knew she hadn't dozed off. She didn't understand it all. Born again? Then he had an altar call and several went forward, and he prayed for them, and then it was over.

"As we depart from God's house today, I would like you to meet some guests of mine," Pastor Paul pointed out to the congregation. "Maria and her daughter, Cat." He waved in their direction, and Cat waved back. "Please make them feel welcome as you go out."

Maria was mortified and grabbed Cat's arm. She'd heard of pastors introducing new attendees, but since he didn't do it earlier in the service, she thought they had escaped recognition. But, it wasn't so bad. Everyone was friendly and wanted them to come back.

Josie introduced Maria and Cat to her parents, and Jake gave Cat a long hug. "She's my friend," he beamed to his parents. Cat gave him a high-five in return.

Josie said she was coming over in a couple days to help Essie with some cleaning, so she hoped to see them both again and have more time to visit. Cat remained silent about her departure date on Tuesday, as she hadn't even told her mother when she was leaving, but Maria should be able to cope better this time since she had so much going on in her life.

Maria and Cat were the last of the congregation to shake Pastor Paul's hand, and he liked it that way. He held Maria's hand in his own and didn't want to let go. "So, how did you like it, Maria? Could you hear all right?"

He was so in hopes that she was more than satisfied and would return next Sunday. She would always have a ride; he would see to that.

"Yes, I heard every word. It was perfect," Maria gushed as she squeezed his hand.

"How about you, Cat? Did you feel at home?" He was so in hopes that the congregation was friendly. He thought they were, but then he had known some of them for years.

"You know, I really did, and of course, we know Josie and Jake, and it was so nice to share a pew with them. Speaking of sharing, we are going out to the buffet to eat, and we were wondering if you'd like to join us." Spur-of-the-moment Cat was full of surprises again!

Maria stared at Cat, and then immediately said, "We are? I mean . . . we are, and we'd love to have your company."

The plans were set to meet in one hour at the Country Kitchen Buffet on Middleford Avenue. That would give Pastor Paul time to tie up loose ends at the church, and Maria was in desperate need of a restroom. Cat found one, and they spruced up and were on their way, stumbling over each other's thoughts and interrupting one another as they talked over the minute details of the morning's events as Cat sped along in her red convertible. She longed to put the top down, but the hairdo would be ruined, and the day had to be perfect for her mother.

Maria was still surprised at the dinner arrangements. "Why didn't you tell me about the buffet plans, Cat? I hope I have enough money with me and my antacids. I hope I brought those. All this excitement could cause a sour stomach."

"Never fear; Cat Woman is here. I have money and Tums."

"Okay, but you just flew through another yellow light," Maria admonished her daughter to no avail. "You might need to save your money for a speeding ticket, and I might need the Tums right now, the way you drive. Just kidding; don't get mad!" She could tell Cat didn't appreciate her advice or her weak attempt at humor.

When Pastor Paul didn't arrive on time, Maria's nerves were as taut as a fishing line with a huge trout on it, but when he pulled in right next to them twenty minutes later, Maria relaxed.

"Sorry for the delay," he said, as he hefted his bulky body out of his sedan. "I got a phone call just as I was leaving the church and had to run back in."

"That's okay; we have all afternoon. I was worried about you, though." Maria just had to say it, and it touched his heart, as did so many other instances throughout the two-hour meal that the three of them shared that Sunday afternoon, and neither Maria or Pastor Paul wanted it to end.

Cat was looking at her watch, and Maria noticed how she was fidgeting.

"Do you have an appointment, Cat?" she asked jokingly.

"As a matter of fact, I do. I told Tony I would meet him this afternoon at the Dairy Queen. Of course, now I'm too full for ice cream. But maybe we should think about going soon."

"If it would make it easier, Cat, I could take your mother home. It won't be out of my way, as if that would matter!" He patted Maria's hand that was resting on the table.

"Oh yeah. You live in the same place; I'd almost forgotten how convenient that makes it." Cat didn't choose her words too well that time, but neither one seemed to make anything out of it and took it at face value.

"Go straight home now, Mother!" Cat winked at Pastor Paul, whose belly shook like the jello he had just consumed.

"She's forgotten who's the mother here," Maria shook her head and grimaced. "She loves to tell me what to do." Then she grabbed Cat's arm and kissed her cheek. "Have a good time, dear, and don't forget your curfew!"

CHAPTER TWENTY-THREE

Pastor Paul and Maria

"These impossible women! How they
do get around us! The poet was right;
Can't live with them or without them."
—Aristophanes

Sunday afternoons were quiet, lazy days at Pear Blossom. The hum of washing machines and dryers in the laundry room or the whir of the elevator sliding to rest on the main floor were often the only intrusions on a silent lobby. Thank goodness, Burton Roop chose to wash his overalls from work on Friday nights! He was one of the few men living in the facility who was still employed, and the zippers and metal snaps and buttons banged and clanged in the laundry room on the last day of the work week without fail as he washed his construction clothes. The Bird Woman swore up and down, but only to herself, that the noise was money swirling around in the dryer, and every week she darted into the laundry room to check as soon as he left, but she never found any coins. She was hoping to add to her collection to store in her freezer. Old or new, she didn't care.

However, that particular Sunday in April, the silence was interrupted by the all-too-familiar wail of sirens, and once again the boxy vehicle pulled up in front of Pear Blossom in the late afternoon. Pastor Paul and Maria just missed witnessing Essie being gently positioned on the gurney and loaded into the ambulance to transport her to the hospital.

In addition, the search had been on for Maria. Michael and Jillian had called most of the morning and into early afternoon looking for her, and as

Pastor Paul parked his silver sedan and escorted Maria in the front door, who should greet them but Maria's son and daughter-in-law.

"Okay, where have you been? We have been calling all day, and where is Cat? We wanted you both to come over for dinner. Who is this man?" Maria felt like a little kid who had been missing and talking to strangers against her parent's wishes.

"Now, don't be rude, Michael. This is Pastor Paul Clairmont, and I've been to church." Michael and Pastor Paul shook hands and looked each other over. "We all had dinner, and now Cat is visiting with Tony—you know, Antonio's son."

Jillian was obviously steamed that they hadn't been notified of the plans, although nothing had been mentioned or set up beforehand. She just felt that most Sundays were reserved for them. "Well, when you didn't answer, we didn't know what to think. We're just glad you are okay." She looked to Michael for agreement, but he and Pastor Paul had walked into the library. A golf match was on television, and Michael had already missed the first few holes. Pastor Paul had no interest in golf, but for the sake of being friendly, he played along with Michael's love of the sport.

They heard a commotion behind them and picked up on a few words. "Passed out right here . . . Eats like a bird . . . No family." Bertha was filling Winnie in on Essie's misfortune.

"Who was it?" Maria asked Jillian, but she didn't know the residents, so Maria quizzed Bertha.

"Essie had a spell, and where have you been? Out with the pastor on a Sunday?"

Bertha was as nosy as the reporters for the *National Enquirer*. If only she had the paparazzi out, she could have seen pictures of Pastor Paul holding Maria's hand as they took the long way home. Bertha continued before Maria could answer. "So, I suppose you two are an item now. I declare, they sure work fast around here." She shook her head in disgust.

"Jealousy does not become you, Bertha, and, in fact, it is a sin." Pastor Paul had stepped out of the library during a commercial and had heard the whole lopsided conversation.

Bertha didn't like that approach one iota. "Look here, Mister. You're preaching to the choir. My father was a pastor, and I've heard all about sin, and yet my father had the audacity to be the biggest sinner and the worst hypocrite in our little country church in Iowa. So, there, how do you like that? So, I'm not one bit jealous. If Maria wants to take her chances, then far be it from me to interfere. In fact, I don't really care." And with that she wheeled out of the lobby and down the west wing to her room as fast as she could spin the tires.

Just then Cat arrived and hurried in the front door with an ice cream cake. Pastor Paul, who was still recovering from Bertha's tirade, could tell it was becoming a family gathering, so he thanked Maria for a wonderful day and excused himself. Maria begged him to join them for dessert, but he assured her by patting his tummy that he was still full from dinner.

The golf tournament was just finishing up, and Michael and Jillian had eaten some small portions of the dessert when Cat sprung another surprise on her mother.

"Since we're all together, I thought I should tell you that Gabby and Gina and I will all be here for Mother's Day. Surprise, Mom, I couldn't keep it a secret any longer!"

"Here? All at once? Mother's Day? Oh, my goodness. How long has it been since we've all been together? Where will you all stay?" The excitement was turning into worry in an instant.

"Don't fret, Mom. We girls, and that includes you, Mom, will have a big slumber party at the Red Lion. I already have a suite reserved for three nights."

"And you'll all be at our house for Mother's Day," Jillian chimed in. "Sorry we don't have more room for you all to stay, but you'll have more fun at the hotel anyway."

Maria was thinking of more problems and negatives. "But what about the cost and the food and how are Gabrielle and Gina going to get here and . . . ?"

"Don't you think we are taking care of all that? Remember, it is Mother's Day. You don't have to do a thing, except show up, and I'm here to tell you, I'll see to that, too, personally! Just mark it on your calendar and look forward to the days in May."

Maria was exhausted by the time Michael and Jillian took off. "Whew! What a day! Church, dinner, Bertha's outburst, poor Essie being carted off, the kids being here, and now the news of more company coming in May . . . I hope I'm up to all of this excitement!" She yawned and kicked her shoes off. "Look at my swollen ankles, Cat. Do you think that is something to worry about?"

"No, just remember to take your water pills tomorrow morning, and that should do the trick. We'll get a mocha, too, and that caffeine, which you didn't have today, will help flush you out. You probably had too much salt today, too. All that ham and scalloped potatoes and good stuff!"

"You should have been a doctor instead of a writer, Cat. You always know what to do."

Cat liked to watch *The Today* Show and it's health-related segments, and she kept up on the various diseases and advancements in medical technology in her reading. "Oh, a lot of it is just common sense," she humbly said, as her mother shuffled off to the bedroom for the night.

"Sweet dreams, dear. I hope you dream about your man." Maria meant well, but she had no idea that Cat had told Tony not to plan on a future with her. "On the morrow I'll tell you what Pastor Paul asked me. I have surprises, too, you know." With that, Maria quickly shut the bedroom door.

As worn out as they both were, sleep didn't come easily for either of them. Maria awakened groggily the next morning, feeling that she had just dozed off and on. Cat couldn't get to sleep, and so she sat on the mattress and wrote in her journal for an hour or so before she could relax. She, too, slept off and on. She hoped she hadn't offended Tony, she was torn between sympathy and dislike for Bertha, she wondered about Essie and her condition, and mostly she wondered what her mother's secret was.

She didn't have to wait long to find out the answer to the latter question. As soon as Maria took her morning's handful of pills, including a diuretic, and Cat had poured the coffee, they sat on the couch to greet the day and each other.

After discussing their night of fitful sleeping and making a few, non-pressing plans for the day, Maria brought up the subject of Pastor Paul herself.

"Well, that was quite a day yesterday, huh? Now, let's first talk about church, Cat. What did you think of his sermon about being a Christian? I didn't understand about being born again, but didn't you love that sentence about how just because you are sitting in church, it doesn't necessarily mean you are a Christian? And then when he added, 'If you sit in your garage all day, that doesn't make you a car,' I thought that was just perfect. I had never thought of Christianity that way, had you, Cat?"

Cat hadn't paid much attention to religion over the years. Her mother had insisted they all attend Sunday school at least through grade school, but since then she always seemed to be busy on Sunday mornings. She hadn't paid much attention to Pastor Paul's sermon either. "Yes, that was quite eloquent;

he has quite a way with words." Cat thought that was a good answer without getting into the theology of the sermon. "And I like the sound of his voice, too," she added. "Is that what attracted you to him?"

"Well, partly, but don't forget the gifts on the doorknob before I ever heard his voice. His words or quotations on the cards were something special. Well, anyway, we had a good day, a nice dinner, and a beautiful ride home. We, . . . um . . . didn't exactly come straight home. We went for a little drive, and he asked me if I would like to go to church with him next Sunday and to dinner, too. I accepted, but then in the middle of the night, it dawned on me that it will be Easter Sunday, and what if Michael and Jillian want to include me in their plans? What will I do? Why do I always get in these messes? I'm so out of practice with all this dating stuff. Cat, help me!"

Cat thought her mother's sudden popularity was hysterically funny, and of course, she had the perfect solution. "The word is *compromise*. You can do both. You can go to church with Pastor Paul and then have dinner with Michael's family. You know—divide your time between the two, and that way no one should have hurt feelings." Cat's devious brain was quietly at work on the sidelines, figuring out how she could put a bug in Jillian's ear about inviting the pastor to dinner, too. "Things work out, Mom. Don't worry."

"But it's one of the things I do best, my dear. Don't deprive me. You always tell me I've made worry an art form!" She gently jabbed Cat in the arm. "Let's have a little breakfast and then get dressed and go to Harry and David's.

"Oh, do you want to become a member of the Fruit of the Month Club like Millie?"

"No, I want to get an idea for something I can take to Jillian's for Easter dinner, if I go."

Cat was pretty sure her mother would be going and with whom; Pastor Paul might not be the Savior himself, but he could help save Maria from depression when Cat went home.

"I just hope I can handle all this excitement and not get run-down or sick. I'll probably be so wound up that my blood will thin out, and it will be zipping through my veins, and the doctor will take me off the Coumadin!"

CHAPTER TWENTY-FOUR

Looking Past the Scars

"If we don't love ourselves,
how can we love anyone else?"
—Joyce Meyers

Essie was one sick, little old gal. Anemia, dehydration, a bladder infection, and the onset of shingles had laid her low, and she was hospitalized for over a week. She couldn't come home until she was stabilized and able to navigate on her own, and she refused to go to rehab or a nursing home. She threatened to check herself out and call a cab.

"There's a little gal who is coming to help me out," she promised the case workers, but when they checked into it, hoping it was someone with nursing abilities, they found out it was Josie Winters doing her senior project. "Well, I tried," Essie consoled herself and resolutely determined she would find another way to get home. That spunk eventually helped her get well enough to return to Pear Blossom.

In the meantime, Josie needed to put in some hours on her project, so with a prayerful heart, she felt she was ready to face Bertha again. Maybe Bertha would soften up, and they could talk about personal things, since now Josie knew about the polio. Maybe Josie could help her see that she needed to be at peace with herself so she could be at peace with others.

Maybe . . .

Josie didn't know where to start on that subject any more than she knew where to start cleaning Bertha's apartment. Her living quarters reflected her life, and from Josie's perspective, they were both a mess. Bertha could tell her where to start sorting and making a way through the clutter, but God would have to guide and direct Josie's path to help clean up Bertha's insecurities.

They got off to a better start. Bertha didn't ask about the little brother, and she patted Josie on the back when she bent over the wheelchair to give Bertha a hug. That's a step, Josie thought, as Bertha showed her where to start sorting.

"I don't like people going through my things, and don't ask any questions about what I have, but these boxes have to be cleaned out and papers thrown away, and as much as I hate to admit it, I need help." She pointed at a stack of boxes in the living room that was beginning to rival the Pyramids. She'd gotten Tony to heave one more on top of the others several times, and in fact, Josie had to get Tony to come in and heave several back down.

Josie passed the papers and pictures and other contents to Bertha who looked each item over carefully before letting Josie *black-bag* it for the *deep six*, as Bertha called their procedure.

The first box went quickly. It contained the most recent bills and medical papers that Bertha thought she should keep, so most of that box was saved. The second box was much more interesting to Josie because it was full of photos. She was bursting with wonder as to who each person was who posed so long ago in the black and white pictures. Most had stern expressions, which caused Josie to ask, "Didn't these people say *cheese*? They all look like they had just sucked on a sour pickle."

Bertha almost laughed, but caught herself. "What was there to smile about? Times were tough. We didn't know if we could afford to get the film developed. But, why am I explaining? You aren't supposed to ask questions, remember?"

"Oh, no, I wasn't trying to be nosy, but I have seen other old pictures and nobody smiled, and I just wondered why not. I thought maybe they thought they looked more dignified that way."

"Those are people I don't even know or didn't like, so there's no use to keep 'em," Bertha said, as she tossed some more in the bag. "They're ancient history to me," she added, resolutely.

As Josie handed Bertha the last picture in the second box, a deer-in-the-headlights look crashed over Bertha's face. She held the picture upside down in both hands for an eternity, and Josie folded her own hands in her lap and waited for Bertha to save it or toss it. Those were the very thoughts circling through Bertha's mind. It had been years since she had seen the man's face, and she wondered why she even had kept the photo. He had hurt her so deeply. Why would she want to look at him again? She'd lost all respect for him. Why should she gaze into those eyes one more time? He had been full of lies and infidelity. Why had he been such a hypocrite?

But, even though she couldn't look at the picture right now, she didn't want to throw it out. Something made her put it aside on the little table by her chair. It was stacked high with junk mail and bills, and the picture, still upside down, rested precariously on the top. She'd think about it later. She wanted to get through one more box.

Josie, of course, could hardly contain her tongue, and her question marks must have been visible as they danced inside of her. She struggled getting down Box Number Three, and as she set it down by Bertha's feet, all of a sudden, Bertha blurted out a question, "Does your dad love you?"

Josie was so astonished at the question and the brusque tone in Bertha's voice with the subject of love that she dropped the papers she had just pulled from the box. *Love* should be said sweetly, and although Josie had never heard any sweetness come out of Bertha's mouth, she thought that she could at least say that word with a light tone and softness to it.

The longer Josie hesitated with her answer, the more unhappy Bertha became. "Didn't you hear me? I asked you if your dad loves you."

"Of course he does. Don't all dads love their kids?" Josie couldn't imagine that they wouldn't, although she had heard kids complain about their dads not paying attention to them, and she'd heard of divorces, where the kids thought it was their fault, and they took the blame.

"Well, yeah, I suppose he would love you because you're perfect, but does he love your brother?" Bertha continued questioning Josie, as she tossed more papers into a black bag.

"Jake? Of course he loves Jake. Everyone loves Jake . . . well, not everyone." Josie knew how Bertha felt about him. "Daddy has to have a lot of patience with Jake, and sometimes it is really hard not to get upset with him, but Jake is so loving himself. He just runs up and throws his arms around everyone, if he thinks they like him. He hears people make fun of him, but it doesn't seem to bother him much. He just finds someone else who loves him. Jake and I know that Daddy loves us because he shows us and tell us all the time. He is a great dad, and he loves Mom a lot, too. We have a pretty good life, even with Jake's problems. God takes good care of us."

"Do we have to bring God into this? All I heard all my life was, 'God does this, and God does that. Praise the Lord. He loves you, Bertha.' Well, He has a funny way of showing it—first I get polio and then my dad, a pastor, ran off with . . . Oh, never mind, I don't want to talk about it. I just don't trust God or men. The church is full of hypocrites. That's why I never go."

Josie knew what hypocrites were. Pastor Paul had preached on it a few years ago. Oh dear, I hope Bertha doesn't think Pastor Paul is a hypocrite, Josie thought, as she handed Bertha some important-looking documents.

Bertha read her mind. "Now, just look at that Pastor Paul. Maria had hardly even gotten her dishes put away in the cupboards when he tried to court her. And you should have seen them, all lovey, dovey on Sunday afternoon. I don't know where they had been, and Maria's family had been looking for her all day."

Josie was pleased to inform the doubter that Maria and Cat had been to the church where Pastor Paul was filling in. "They sat in our pew," Josie beamed with enthusiasm. "I guess I don't really know what a hypocrite is if it's wrong for two people to like each other. I've never really seen them together, you know, because he was up in front preaching, but I bet they are cute."

"Cute? At their age?" Bertha snorted and shook her head. "I wouldn't trust him just because he's a pastor. He just moved in too fast with Maria."

"That's why. He has to hurry because they are old and might run out of time." Josie giggled at her little joke, but Bertha could see no humor in it whatsoever.

She moved her wheelchair, and in trying to toss a letter on top of the picture on the table, she knocked the picture to the floor right-side up, and as Josie reached out to pick it up, Bertha screamed, "Turn it over! I don't want to see it!"

Josie looked at the picture and then at Bertha. She was staring at the picture when Bertha reached out her short, stubby fingers and snatched it away. "Don't look at him, and don't tell me I look just like him. I've heard that all my life, too! I don't want to look like my dad!"

"Oh, that's your dad? You *do* look like him. Wow! He was cool looking."

"Yeah, well, the church secretary thought so, too, apparently. I thought I told you I didn't want to talk about him! I've told you far too much, and I don't want you going out into that lobby and telling all my secrets to those old, gossipy women. None of them even like me, and they're all nuttier than a fruitcake." Bertha was as agitated as a washing machine on an extra spin cycle.

"Calm down, Bertha. I'm not going to tell anyone what you told me." Josie didn't know what a person looked like when they were having a stroke or what to do, so she tried to change the subject in case Bertha was working up to one. Maybe she should try again to tell Bertha that God really does love her or that maybe the residents don't like her too well because she doesn't seem to like herself. This is pretty heavy duty stuff, Josie thought. She didn't know if she could handle it.

After a pause, Josie decided to try something her mother had told her. "If we let other people drive us nuts, maybe it's because we don't like ourselves. It's hard to get along with other people if we don't even like ourselves. I think even Jake likes himself. Do you like yourself, Bertha?"

"Now, why would I like myself—this old, crippled up body? Have to sit in this ugly chair all the time, can't do anything or go anywhere. I think that was a pretty stupid question, Missy. It's not much of a life, and people make me so mad! Like you're doing right now!"

Josie could relate to that in Jake's life, and she shared her thoughts with Bertha. "Jake used to get mad when people made fun of him, but somehow after we prayed a lot with him, he seems to be more at peace about the way he looks and talks. He doesn't get so frustrated when he can't do something or someone says something to hurt him. So now he seems to be happier with himself and he's able to give that love away."

Bertha was determined to take it the wrong way. "Are you comparing me with that Mongoloid?"

"Down Syndrome, Bertha, and yeah, in a way I am. You are both sort of crippled. His body is imperfect, too. He can run and play ball, but not like normal kids, and like you are trapped in that wheelchair, he is trapped with a mind that doesn't work like other kids his age. But he just accepts it and goes on now, since we've prayed about it."

Bertha had heard enough for one day. "He just doesn't know any better, but I do. At least my mind works."

"See, there is something to like about yourself." Josie thought that she had said enough for one session. She hoped that leaving Bertha with that positive thought might give her something to think about for a few days, and in all sincerity as she went out the door, Josie said, "By the way, Bertha, I just want you to know that I really like you."

"Hmmph," Bertha grunted at the door that was closing. "Well, at least I do have my mind," she repeated the thought out loud to herself. "I can still think straight, and I know what is going on around here when nobody else does. I know the rules and how to enforce them. Why, I could run this place! And I can still balance my checkbook, too, if I could ever find it!"

PEAR BLOSSOM RESIDENT'S BULLETIN BOARD
EASTER SUNDAY POTLUCK SUNDAY, APRIL 17 1:00 P.M.
(This will be the potluck for the month)
BAKED HAM supplied by Oscar and Otis:
Everybody else just bring whatever!! No sign-up sheet this time.
MOTHERS DAY
May 14 ENJOY WITH YOUR FAMILY
OR ADOPT A FAMILY FOR THE DAY!

*   *   *

SOMETHING TO THINK ABOUT:

The activities director (me—Betty) is thinking about us having a dog birthday party later on in May or June. Let me know what you think (I'm sure you will), but only if you are interested. I don't want to hear negatives! Dogs like to have fun, too!

ATTENTION:
Coffee cans needed for a friend of mine.
Contact Blanche

BIRTH ANNOUNCEMENT:
Be sure to congratulate Emily on the birth of her new great granddaughter, Ava. She (Ava, not Emily) weighed 8 lbs.

FOR SALE:
(Perpetually)
Old clothes; Fancy dresses and blouses; Boas, gowns, high heels, hats.
No slacks.
See Millie or call 647-0177

FOR SALE BY OWNER
One pair women's slacks
Size 14; They are too long in the Crouch. Call: Winnie 647 5555

CHAPTER TWENTY-FIVE

Mother's Day Weekend

"Many daughters have done virtuously,
But thou excellent them all."
—Proverbs 31:29

Easter Sunday without Cat. She had gone back home to Hillsboro on Tuesday and although Maria missed her, she was too busy to sit around and mope. She attended church with Pastor Paul on Easter, and then they both were invited to an Easter barbeque at Michael and Jillian's.

"That was awfully nice of them to include me," Pastor Paul remarked to Maria on Wednesday of the following week. Maria was attending his Bible study each week, and although she didn't always understand the lesson, at least she was making an effort, for his sake, and she did accept Jesus as her savior!! "You're born again, Maria." Pastor Paul was ecstatic

"As long as you don't make me read aloud or answer any questions, I will go," Maria had forewarned him. "You know, I don't see too well."

Pastor Paul had promised not to embarrass her. "Just sit and listen and take it all in. God will bless your heart. It blesses *my* heart that you are coming to hear God's word."

Maria tried to listen, but all she could think about was his voice and his laughter. He liked to start Bible study with a joke, just like he did with his Sunday sermon, and she concentrated hard so she could remember the story and the punch line, but she never had been good at jokes and she was worse now. Often she would ask him afterwards to repeat it again for her. She loved to see him enjoy his own stories, and that belly laugh in itself was worth the replay of the joke.

Rumor had it that Pastor Paul and Maria were becoming an item, and by the time Mother's Day weekend rolled around, the story, circulating like an oscillating fan, was that they were engaged. Sarah and Jess were still seeing each other, and Oscar played up to Millie every chance he could get. Antonio had given up on Millie. He was just too old and too tired to try any more. Maria caught his fancy, but he was too slow to catch her.

"You can have Millie, old boy," he told Oscar. "She's too much for me!"

Oscar was still such a novice at courting, but at least his dandruff was better, and his wardrobe was less dismal and boring. He even wore a brightly colored Hawaiian shirt a few times that he had gotten at Goodwill. He couldn't get Old, Blue Otis to lighten up, and so he still wore his postal colors that he'd worn to work for so many years. "I have no one to dress up for like you do," he moaned to Oscar.

But no one seemed to pay as much attention to the other couples as they did to Maria and Pastor Paul. Bertha was the lookout for when they went out and when they came in, and like a mother hen, she made sure he went to his own apartment each night. The next day the gaggle of geese lined up for her report, and the rumor mill spun out another story.

But they didn't care. They weren't doing anything sinful, and they knew the busybodies had nothing better to do with their time.

"Isn't it fun to provide some activity and intrigue for those poor old souls who have nothing else to do?" Maria felt like she was really contributing something worthwhile. "Ah, sweet mystery of life," she told Pastor Paul, who by now had become just Paul to her. "What will they have to chatter about next week when my girls come for Mother's Day? I'll be gone to that hotel."

"I'm not as worried about the gossips finding something else to do as I am worried about what I will do all weekend," Paul said sadly. "It will be the longest weekend of my life—four days, you say?"

"Oh, come on; it won't be so bad; you'll get to meet my girls. We'll get together somehow, somewhere. In fact, come to think about it, Gina and Gabby will come here to see my apartment, and you can meet them then. We aren't going to hole up in that hotel the whole time, I hope."

"Did you say you have another daughter in Connecticut? Is she coming?"

"Yes, you mean Laura. No, she can't get away. She's a registered nurse and her schedule is hectic. Maybe someday before I die, she'll get to come out west again."

Pastor Paul didn't like her talking about her demise. "Well, let's live it up while we can, Maria. How would you like to watch those Gaither videos tonight?"

Maria was getting bolder. "My apartment or yours?" And so their romance continued.

*   *   *

Gina arrived from Santa Barbara, and Gabby flew in from Spokane within a couple hours of each other. Cat had returned to Middleford in time to pluck them both from the airport. They decided they wanted to see where their mama lived before they settled in for the weekend at the hotel, so Cat zipped them through the yellow lights and across town to Pear Blossom. Gina was used to speeding over the California freeways, so Cat's driving was fine with her. Gabby was thankful that the streets of Middleford were so smooth, unlike the potholes that swallowed up her car on the city streets of Spokane.

Maria was waiting on the bench out in front of the "home" with Pastor Paul, when her three girls arrived, and of course, the chinwaggers inside were on the alert to cast their approval or dismay over her daughters. Maria warned them as they got out of the car that they would be pounced upon like a cat attacks a mouse by the gossips inside.

"Well, our Cat can pounce right back," Gabby giggled as she jabbed Gina in the ribs. "Isn't this already like old times, sis?"

Gina was the most serious one of all of Maria's girls, but she laughed and agreed with Gabby. "It sounds pretty dangerous around here. Are you safe to be living here, Mama?"

"Oh, their bark is worse than their bite. They just don't have anything better to do with their time," Maria said.

"Did you hear that, Cat? Now, they're barking! Is this a pet store?"

"No, but they are going to have a dog birthday party, maybe next month," Cat said. "See, that's why I called them *mixed nuts!*"

The hilarity went on all weekend, and they all had a wonderful time together. They went to a play, *Shirley Valentine,* at Bear Creek Community College, the girls took Maria to a spa where she got her first-ever massage and a badly needed pedicure, and they shopped at Carlotta's in the mall.

"Now don't tell Pastor Paul that I'm out on the town and drinking Bloody Marys," Maria begged her daughters on Saturday night after the play. They stopped in at the bar in the hotel to listen to some music before turning in.

"Oh, you only had one, and it had so many veggies skewered on the top that it looked more like a salad than a drink," Gabby reassured her. "Besides, we already met him yesterday, so doubt that we'll see him again. Oh dear, we don't have to go to church tomorrow, do we?"

"No, I'll give up the Lord for one Sunday to be with you girls," Maria said demurely. "But, did you like him? Pastor Paul, I mean." She wanted to make sure just one more time.

"Yes, he seemed just perfect, Mom. But, you know me, I've never been too good a judge of character. Two husbands later, and I'm still not sure if I have the right one." Gina was never sure of herself, and her indecision drove Maria crazy.

"We think he is cute, don't we?" Cat looked to Gabby for agreement and got it. "You make a perfect couple. We all agree on that!" Cat delivered the jury's decision with unanimous applause.

Pastor Paul, meanwhile, had a miserable weekend. He wasn't sure if it was just loneliness or if he was coming down with something. He felt just a little off-center all day Saturday, and Sunday morning was even worse. A dull pain was lingering in his back as he struggled to the church to greet all the mothers and children and deliver the expected Mother's Day sermon.

By the time the service was over, the pain had traveled clear through his back to his abdomen. He turned down several dinner invitations, including one from Josie and her family. Smiling and being polite at a Sunday dinner table was the last thing he wanted to do. All he could think about on the drive home was to get to his apartment and to lie down.

While Maria was having a lovely dinner with her daughters at Michael and Jillian's house, Pastor Paul's pain was getting worse by the hour. Finally, around 4:30 in the afternoon, he called for an ambulance. There were several folks in the lobby, and as the medics wheeled him out, he raised his head and mumbled through the pain, "Don't tell Maria!"

"What did he say?" Millie asked, as she looked around the lobby. But no one seemed to have heard him or knew what was going on.

"We'd better call Maria," Sarah advised, thinking that if something ever happened to Jess, she would want to know immediately.

Millie thought that was a good idea, "But, where is she? I haven't seen her for days."

"No, it's NOT a good idea. Didn't you just hear him say not to call her?" Bertha's antennae had been on high-voltage, and she had heard it all. "It's probably just spring fever or puppy love or whatever old people get when they think they're in love. It's probably nothing." Bertha's doctorate degrees in both medicine and affairs of the heart were non-existent, but that didn't stop her from expressing her know-it-all opinion with full authority. "She's with her girls for Mother's Day, so just leave her alone."

Oscar was just pulling up out in front, and as Millie tripped out the door in her high heels, she turned and said, "Bertha has spoken, and although I couldn't hear what she said, I guess we'd better leave well enough alone. She's always right! Ta Ta, girls! See you at the Dairy Queen!"

"Is that the only place she and Oscar ever go?" Sarah wondered aloud.

Bertha thought so and said sarcastically, "Yes, they share one banana split. Now, isn't that romantic?"

"It is if you're in love. Jess and I sometimes share a chocolate sundae, but you know, with all my lactose intolerance problems, it just doesn't set too well with me, so I let him eat most of it. Oh, here he comes now. He was supposed to get me some Prilosec; I hope he didn't forget."

Bertha turned her wheels to travel to her apartment. "Let me know if you hear anything about Pastor Paul," she called over her shoulder to Sarah, "but don't tell Maria."

*   *   *

"It's your gall bladder," Dr. Woolf assured Paul Clairmont, after several hours in the ER, a shot to help the pain, and an ultrasound that showed several stones. "Now that the pain has subsided, here are your options. You can go home and hope it never happens again, or you can call tomorrow and schedule surgery. I would advise the latter. Rich foods could trigger another attack. Any questions? I don't mean to be blunt and in a hurry, but I guess you can hear that woman screaming behind that curtain over there." Dr. Woolf shook Paul's hand. "Think about it, okay?"

Paul didn't have to think long and hard. The pain had been like an arrow shot through from back to front, and he hoped to never experience that again. The next morning he called and made arrangements to see a surgeon and schedule gall bladder surgery. Now, they'll have to get an interim pastor for the interim pastor, he thought. That bothered him more than anything—that, and having to tell Maria. He reassured himself with the thoughts that at least he had her in his life, and she could help him get through it all. It could bring them even closer together, or it could backfire, and she might decide she didn't want to take care of a sick, old man. One thing was for sure: it would delay his plans.

The weekend had gone all too quickly for Maria. She accompanied Cat and the girls to the airport and waved goodbye with tears in her eyes as her two daughters went through security on Monday morning. "Isn't that ridiculous that they have to take off their shoes! Do my daughters look like terrorists?" she lamented to Cat.

"Everyone is a suspect these days. Look over there at that old lady in the wheelchair with the fuzzy, permed hair. She must be in her 80's, and they are waving their magic wand over her, looking for who-knows-what. She sure looks suspicious to me!" Cat tried to humor her mother, but it fell on deaf ears. She put her arm around Maria and steered her toward the door.

Maria was wiping the tears from her cheeks. "Yeah, let's get out of here and go home. I am just exhausted! But, Cat, wasn't it fun all being together? It meant so much to me, and thank you for arranging it all. I'll never forget it as long as I live!"

"We'll do it again, unless you run off with Pastor Paul," Cat teased.

"We'll do it again even if I do run off with Paul, oh . . . what am I saying? I'm not running off with him!"

CHAPTER TWENTY-SIX

The Proposal

"If only, when one heard that old age was coming,
One could bolt the door, answer, "Not at home"
And refuse to meet him!"
—Kokinshu (Ancient Poetry)

Pondering over a cup of coffee and the *Guidepost* magazine, Paul was anxious to see Maria, but not happy about breaking the news to her of his ailment and his impending surgery. "Worry is the darkroom where negatives are developed," he read, and he nodded his head and bowed it in prayer. He talked to God every day, but it was usually of an intercessory nature, prayers for others who needed help in one form or another. Today he needed God's comfort for himself.

As he was praying, he heard a gentle tapping on the door. It can't be Jesus wanting in; he'd opened that door to Him long ago. No, there it was again, and he quickly ended his prayer and answered the door. There stood Maria. It was the first time she had been bold enough to come to his apartment uninvited, and she was a sight for his tired, old eyes. His hand flew to his side where the pain had been just in case the richness of her beauty caused another attack.

"Oh, my dear, do come in." And as the door closed, he grabbed her and kissed her full on her painted lips. "I'm sorry, but you have no idea how I've needed you and missed you," he apologized profusely, as beads of sweat formed on his brow.

"Is something wrong, Paul? You look so pale!" Maria held his face in her two hands with concern filling her heart. "Tell me what is wrong," she pleaded.

"Let's sit over here, and I'll tell you what happened," and they sat on the couch while he told her of his horrible weekend—the pain, the time in the hospital, and the diagnosis. He had promised himself he would be blasé about it and act in control to free her from worry, but remembering that terrible pain as he told her about it, upset him all over again. "It was just so horrible. I thought I was going to die and never see you again, Maria."

"Why didn't someone try to get hold of me? I would have come right away." Maria didn't know who to blame, but one of her friends should have called the hotel or Michael's, she thought.

"I didn't want to spoil your weekend, so I told them not to call you, my dear. I wanted you to have a good time. Did you? Oh, I have been babbling on about myself and haven't even asked about your girls and your Mother's Day. Talk to me, Maria, and tell me all about it."

She told him every detail, except for the part about her drinking a Bloody Mary, and the stories seemed to calm him down. The color came back into his cheeks, and his belly laugh assured her that she was good medicine.

They made plans for the surgery and the recovery. Thankfully, it would be the easy kind and not the big slice through the abdomen that Maria had endured twenty-some years ago. She had never shown anyone her scar, and she surely wasn't going to bare her wound to Pastor Paul, so she was thankful that he took her word that it was long and ugly.

He was just about ready to bring up another subject, a subject he had put off long enough, when Maria announced that she must be going because Cat was still around.

"She'll be leaving tomorrow morning, and I promised her I wouldn't be long. What time is it, anyway?"

"Too late . . . I mean, it's getting late and I bet you are both tired," he said, as he glanced at his watch. "We'll talk again tomorrow. Oh, I am so glad you are back!"

"Me too, for several reasons," Maria stifled a yawn.

"May I have one more little kiss before you go, please?"

"Well, since you said *Please*, I guess so," she teased and puckered up. "Now, let's both get some rest, and I'll check on you first thing in the morning, and Paul, please call me if you need anything, do you promise?"

"I promise, since you said *Please*. Now, don't worry; I'll be fine. Tell Cat good-bye for me."

Cat was napping on the couch when Maria returned to her apartment. She tried to tip-toe around and unpack her suitcase, but Cat woke up the minute she unzipped her bag.

"Oh, I must have dozed off. What took you so long? Was the good pastor proposing?"

"Cat, why are you trying to get me married off so fast? No, he was not proposing. He's sick. He was sick all weekend, and nobody bothered to call me. He has to have surgery, Cat. Isn't that sad?" Maria wrung her hands and plopped down on the couch. "I feel so sorry for him."

"So, what is his problem? Did he say? If not, it's probably his prostate. Men have problems there, you know, and they don't like to talk about it."

"Oh, Cat, you sound just like Bertha with all of her advice. Yes, I do know about men and their problem areas. No, this is his gall bladder, and it has to come out."

Cat reassured her mother with some more medical knowledge. "It's a piece of cake nowadays, unlike the way you had it done. Remember the pain and the morphine and all?"

"Ah, yes, I remember it well, Cat. You had to come and help me. Well, I'll be here to help Paul, in whatever way I can. It's harder to heal the older we get. See, I know some things about our bodies, too," she smugly replied.

Cat didn't want their last day together to end with hurtling snide remarks back and forth, so she changed the subject. "How about if I wash some clothes?"

"No, I'll do the dirty wash; you plug the wrong machine with quarters, remember? You are still two quarters short of a full load, my dear! Come on; let's sort 'em and go do it."

Maria had so much on her mind with Paul's pending surgery that the waves of depression didn't consume her every thought and minute as before. She missed Cat and all her girls, but Paul wanted to spend as much time with her as he could, "before I go under the knife," as he called his surgery. "One never knows what might happen."

Each morning that week Maria found a little card and note on her door from Paul. At least now she knew who was pursuing her, but that didn't ruin the intrigue; she was still excited to check every morning for the newest love note.

The one that really got to her was a card tied to the doorknob on Thursday morning:

"Darling, I am growing old,
Silver threads among the gold
Shine upon my brow today;
Life is fading fast away."

At the end he added his own personal note: "Maria, can you come to my apartment as soon as possible. We need to talk! Love, Paul"

Broken with worry, Maria hurried through her morning routine and was dashing, as best she could, through the lobby to Paul's apartment when she remembered that she'd forgotten to take her pills. Or had she taken them? She was muttering so loudly to herself that Essie heard her.

"I always take my Coumadin at night, and it helps me sleep better. You should try it, Maria, and another thing I like to do is write down every time I pee!" She smiled and nodded at Maria.

"Well, I'm not into keeping a journal and especially not of my bodily functions." Maria brushed past her in her hurry to get to Paul's apartment. "Excuse me, but I have to go."

"What, you have vertigo?" Essie shouted, as Maria hurried down the hall, shaking her head. "That's worse than having *authoritis,* which I have, along with all my other troubles."

Paul was looking up and down the hall, and he could smell Maria's Giorgio cologne and could hear her humming *The Tennessee Waltz* before she came into full view. She was almost running.

"Hey, slow down. Where's the fire?" Bertha popped out of her apartment, and Maria had to dodge her wheelchair. "Oh, it's just him," Bertha said with disgust when she spotted Paul. "He can wait. You don't have to be in such a rush! Men aren't worth it."

"Here she comes, Miss America!" Paul began singing in his strong tenor voice when Maria got closer. "Hi, honey," he whispered in her ear as she fell into his arms. "Are you all right? He could feel her heart pounding next to his, and she was literally gasping for air.

"Yes, I'm fine, but what about you? Your note sounded so urgent. Are you sick?"

"No, I'm fine, well, everything considered. I just want to talk to you. Sorry if I upset you, and you thought I was dying or something." Paul escorted her to the couch. "Want some coffee?"

"I'd really just rather have a glass of cold water, if you don't mind, Paul. I'm all dried out!"

As Paul handed her the tall glass of ice water with a lemon slice in it just like she loved, he said, "That reminds me of a joke. Have you heard the one about the old lady at the flower show? It's not one I could tell at church or Bible study, but it is funny. I hope it won't offend you."

Maria felt relieved that Paul seemed so chipper and well enough to entertain her with his humor. "If I've heard it, I don't remember it. I can never

remember them and can't tell 'em, so go ahead." She knew how he loved to start any conversation or lesson or sermon with a joke.

"Okay. Two old ladies were sitting on a park bench outside the local town hall where a flower show was in progress. One leaned over and said, 'Life is so boring; we never have any fun any more. For $5.00, I'd take my clothes off and streak through that stupid flower show!'

'You're on!' said the other old lady, holding up a $5.00 bill.

As fast as she could, the first little old lady fumbled her way out of her clothes and, completely naked, streaked through the front door of the flower show. Waiting outside, her friend soon heard a huge commotion inside the hall, followed by loud applause. The naked lady burst through the door surrounded by a cheering crowd.

'What happened?' asked her waiting friend.

'I won 1st prize as BEST DRIED ARRANGEMENT!'"

Paul could hardly finish the punch line before he collapsed in gales of laughter. His deep belly laugh that Maria usually enjoyed worried her. "Be careful, Paul. What if your gall stones come loose and move around? Oh dear. Try to control yourself! That *was* funny, though."

"Well, you aren't laughing much. I hope it wasn't too offensive," Paul expected more of an enjoyable reaction.

"I am just so worried about you! Is that what you enticed me down here to tell me?"

"Were you expecting more?" Paul hoped so, and he didn't really give Maria a chance to answer. He slowly arose from the couch and walked over to the small table in front of the window where a vase with one red rose graced a white doily. Picking up the vase, he returned to the couch and Maria. "This is for you. A red rose to show my love for you," and he handed her the vase.

"Oh, Paul, it's my favorite flower." She buried her nose in its petals and although her sense of smell had gone the way of her dark, brown hair, she told him she loved the fragrance.

"I have something else for you, too, Maria." He pulled a straight-backed chair over from the little dining area and placed it squarely in front of her and sat down. He took her hands in his. "I don't think I could get down on one knee any more, and if I could, you'd have to help me back up, but I do want to ask you something. I've wanted to ask you this for several weeks, but now the time is right. I've prayed about this every day and hoped I wasn't pursuing you too quickly or with too much fanfare. God told me that we are both getting old, and time is of the essence, and so now, Maria, will you marry me? Whew! There, I finally said it!" He rubbed his forehead in relief

and looked into her eyes with question marks dancing between them. "I'm sorry, but I don't have an engagement ring yet. I thought I should pop the question first, and we can pick out rings together."

"Oh, my goodness! Cat was right. She thought you were going to propose, but I pooh-poohed it, and now here you've done it. Oh dear!"

"Is it *that* bad?" Paul was taken aback with her discouraging comments. "Have I been too forward? Maybe I acted too quickly. Oh, my dear, I'm so sorry!"

"Oh, no, Paul, I just really wasn't expecting it. Why would you want me? I'm an old lady!"

"Well, look at me; I'm an old man. We should be an old couple together! I want to beg you to say 'yes', but I won't. Just please think about it, Maria. You must know that I love you."

"Oh, Paul, I do know that, and I have loved all your little poems of love and the flowers and the candy. I am just so surprised that anyone would even look at me at my age, let alone fall in love with this wrinkled up old face, half-blind eyes, and ailments that you don't even know about and don't want to. I just never expected anyone to fall for me ever again!" Maria wiped her eyes that no longer could hold back a flood of tears.

"There, there now. I'm no beauty myself. Old, fat, bald, and now I am even running around with a bad gall bladder. Time takes its toll, and we just have to thank God for every day and hold onto His hand, and I hope hold onto each other's, but, I won't pressure you; just think about it."

Ten seconds later Maria responded, "Okay, I've thought about it."

CHAPTER TWENTY-SEVEN

A Glimmer of Hope

"When the Lord does it,
you don't have to work so hard on it."
—Tom Van Der Ende

Josie Winters was winding down her junior year of high school, and her counselor recommended that she take the summer off from her senior project at Pear Blossom. Josie was far ahead of her other class members in fulfilling the requirements that were due a year away, and her advisor was sure she must need a break from those "old people."

Just when I was making progress with Bertha, Josie thought, but to appease her advisor, she agreed. Bertha might need me, though. Her place is still a mess! I could just go and help her on a friendly basis and not as a student, Josie decided. God wants me to keep trying!

When Josie talked to Sherrie about it, the administrator was surprised. She hadn't realized that their last workday had gone better, and she agreed that Bertha could use the help. Josie didn't tell her that Bertha had opened up a little and let her see a crack in her heart that needed to be healed. "We are starting to get along better," was all that Josie offered.

Bertha was shocked when she opened the door to find both Sherrie and Josie standing in the hall. "What's going on? What has happened that I missed?" She tried to look up and down the hallway, but they were in her way. "Did the ambulance come again? Oh, I bet I know; Paul and Maria eloped!"

Sherrie was quick to dissuade her guesses of adventures in the facility. "No, no, nothing happened at all. You didn't miss a thing, for once, Bertha. Josie

just wondered if she could help you some more—you know—with sorting and cleaning or whatever. School is almost out for the summer, so she'll have more free time, plus she is free right now."

Bertha snorted, "You mean you don't have a summer job? I think all people your age should be working. You are just too lazy."

Josie had a very busy schedule, even in the summer, but, of course, Bertha didn't know that and just judged her on other's lifestyles. Bible School was coming up next week, and she was helping with that, and then she would be starting her new job at Beans on Broadway.

Bertha's response when she told her of her job was typical: "Oh well, anyone can make coffee." Josie didn't argue with her, and as Sherrie left them alone, they started sorting through boxes again. Old bills and receipts from fifteen years ago weren't very exciting or worthwhile saving, so the black garbage bags filled up quickly. Josie looked around furtively for the picture of Bertha's dad that had upset her so much the time before, but it was nowhere in sight.

"We are making headway, aren't we?" Bertha mentioned the obvious, but at least it was positive. "It will be nice to have more room in here. Sometimes I almost get claustrophobic with all these piles of junk around. How many more boxes are there? Maybe we can get them done today, if you don't dilly dally. Come on; get a move on, girl."

"Just three more, it looks like," Josie said, as she lifted another box of papers and placed it near Bertha's wheelchair. "These look like letters, maybe love letters, so I won't read them. You sort them." Josie moved her chair back and sat down.

Bertha actually laughed, but it was a nervous, sarcastic outburst of dismay. "Now, who do you think would write me love letters? You must be kidding." She pursed her lips and scowled as she rummaged through the letters. "Oh, I did have a boy friend once, but he never wrote any letters. He was a just a little guy, a jockey. I think he loved horses more than he loved me. My family didn't like him, and that's why I did. But he rode too many winners and got the big head and rode off into the sunset. Oh, why am I talking about this? That was a long time ago, and it doesn't matter!" She continued to sift through the envelopes, and Josie was just dying to know who had written to her.

"Nosy, aren't you?" Bertha could see her straining her eyes and craning her neck.

"Okay, I'll tell you. These are letters I found that my dad wrote to that secretary, and they are love letters that he never mailed. Why not? I don't know, but nevertheless, they make me sick! Some are letters that she wrote

to him, and they make me want to vomit! He left them when he ran off with her, and then he didn't even marry her; he dumped her in the trash just like he'd dumped us!"

"Then why did you save the letters?" Josie's eyes swelled with wonder. "Why didn't you throw them away or burn them?" This was all too much for a young, naive, Christian girl to take in.

Bertha shrugged her shoulders. "Oh, I wanted to burn them, but I didn't have a fireplace, and I couldn't find a burning barrel, and then I thought maybe I could blackmail him with 'em, but then I finally decided that if I kept them around, I could hate him just that much more!"

"And that was your dad that did all that, and he was a pastor?" Josie was utterly shocked.

"That's what he called himself. I call him a liar and a hypocrite, and the poorest excuse for a dad in the whole world, and I will hate him until the day I die and then some!"

Bertha's anger was hot enough to burn the whole box of letters right in front of Josie. Her entire body was shaking, and perspiration was dripping from her brow. Hot, burning anger!

Josie jumped up and got her a glass of cold water and a Kleenex and tried to calm her down.

Josie thought of things to say, but should she? Would they just make Bertha more upset? She didn't seem to be in any mood to accept anything scriptural or spiritual. Maybe Josie should just keep quiet and console her and try to love her.

"What's the matter, girl? Cat got your tongue? I shocked you, didn't I? Well, even a nice girl like you has to learn that there are evil people in the world and not to trust everybody. So, there, I've taught you a lesson." Bertha was in control again.

"Yeah, I am kind of speechless. My dad is so cool that it's hard to believe that could happen to you. But, even with the bad people in the world, we should love them, even if we don't like everything they do. You know, love the sinner, but hate the sin. I guess it would be really hard to forgive your dad, but maybe you could try?"

"Josie Winters, I could really be mad at you now for trying to preach to me, but you know what? I'm not. You are wise beyond your years, and someday you should be a missionary. Not a pastor; I don't believe in women pastors, but a missionary. Even I, a tired, cranky, spiteful old woman, know you are right. I've heard it all before. But it's not in me to be so forgiving. I found out a long time ago that no one will look out for poor, old crippled Bertha.

I have to look out for myself, and that means being tough on the outside, opinionated, and even domineering. See, I know how I come across. I have to be in charge. It's the only way I can deal with life. There! Did I shock you again?" Bertha sighed, a long audible sigh that settled her chest and relieved some of the tension.

Hard-hearted Bertha, a softy underneath all that bluster and critical demeanor? Yes, Josie was shocked! She always took people at face-value—what you see is the way they are, period, but *maybe* Bertha could learn to forgive and learn to like herself. Oh, what a senior project Josie had!

CHAPTER TWENTY-EIGHT

Sarah's Loose Tongue

"A closed mouth gathers no feet."
—Anon

"Can you believe it's June already?" Sarah asked Maria, as she flipped through the summer issue of *Good Housekeeping*. "Didn't we just have Valentine's Day?" They were sitting in the waiting room of Bear Creek Community Hospital waiting for Pastor Paul's surgeon to walk into view and tell them that the gall bladder surgery was over and all was well.

"Yes, time just speeds by, except for times like this when you want it to hurry up."

Maria checked her watch again as she'd been doing every minute for the last hour. "That doctor should be coming any minute. I am a nervous wreck. Paul said to just put it in God's hands, but I firmly believe that sometimes He needs my help!" Her furrowed worry lines showed her fears.

"Oh, you are so funny, Maria, but I agree. I am a big worrier, too. My biggest problem now is my feet. My big toe on my right foot . . . Oh, look, here comes a doctor, I think."

Maria was greatly relieved that she didn't have to hear about Sarah's big toe on her right foot, although it wasn't Paul's surgeon. It was a doctor for the other party in the room, but he captured Sarah's interest, and she strained to hear what he had to say. She could only catch snatches of his diagnosis, but Maria was thankful it gave her something to do. She did appreciate Sarah's companionship, though, on a day like this. She had even decided to tell Sarah her big news, when she could get the chance at the right time.

Nobody else, except Cat, knew that Maria had accepted Paul's proposal. They hadn't set a date, and she wasn't wearing an engagement ring, so it was still hush-hush, which Maria and Paul knew was driving the residents crazy. She and Paul were seen together often, and whispers were turning into bold questions. They both thought it was fun to have a secret, and they evaded the questions like a kid who gets caught with his hand in the cookie jar. Bertha, of course, was the main interrogator, but she seemed more interested than just being bossy and nosy. Paul and Maria had commented several times to each other that it seemed odd that she wasn't so grumpy and disapproving, and they wondered if she was sick or something.

"No, maybe I'm just jealous. Did you ever think of that?" A surprising reply when they had asked recently of her health, but then one never knew what to expect from Bertha. She would be the last one they would tell of their engagement.

When Sarah had finished eavesdropping and was so disappointed that she couldn't pick up on the doctor's report to the family nearby, Maria grabbed the chance to share her big news.

"I have something you might be interested in hearing, Sarah." Maria was as excited as a young bride. "Now, you can't tell anyone. Nobody knows yet, so if I hear it gets out, I'll know who blabbed."

Scooting to the very edge of her chair, Sarah clasped her hands. "Oh, tell me. I won't breathe a word of it, I promise! Is it what I think it is? You've decided to go to Italy with Cat? Oh, I'm so excited for you! I hope you get to go to Tuscany. Remember that calendar I had, Maria, of Tuscany? It must be so beautiful there. Oh, look, here comes another doctor."

Before Maria could straighten Sarah out and cancel the Tuscany trip idea, Paul's doctor strode into the room. "It's over," he said hurriedly, as he stood squarely in front of Maria. "No problems; very routine surgery. He can go home tomorrow. Any questions?"

Maria's relief came out in tears. "Oh, bless you, doctor! I am so relieved!"

"No questions, then? Okay. Just let him rest a few more minutes, and then you can go see him." He reached out and shook Maria's hand, nodded at Sarah, and turned and marched down the hall.

By the time Paul went home the next day in a taxi with Maria by his side, it was all over Pear Blossom that Maria was going off to Italy with her daughter and leaving him to recuperate alone. Maria had been so eager to be with Paul in his hospital room that she had politely dismissed Sarah without clearing up the misinformation of the trip, or making her big announcement of future plans, and Sarah had called Jess to come and pick her up.

"You know, the daughter named Kitten, who drives that red convertible," Essie said to Emily in the lobby the next morning. "She is taking Maria to Italy, all expenses paid."

Emily steered clear of gossip and dissension, but somehow Essie cornered her by the mailboxes, and Emily had to correct her. "I believe her name is Cat," she said, as sweetly as honey dripping from the jar. "She's a nice gal and such a good daughter to Maria. I'm happy for them."

"Guess she doesn't care as much about Pastor Paul as it appears, if she's going off and leaving that sick, old man. Maybe there's hope for me yet with him," Millie flipped her beach towel over her leathered shoulder, as she bent over to search her mailbox. She was in her bikini and on her way out to the back patio to "catch some rays," as she called her summer tanning sessions.

"But I thought you liked Oscar," the Bird Woman twittered. "I am so confused!"

"Aren't we all?!" Winnie chimed in. "I thought you secretly liked Antonio, Millie."

"Oh, anyone will do. It doesn't matter, just so I have a man!" She cooed and preened.

Otis, whose hearing was perfect, heard it all from the balcony. He was leaning over the railing, as he liked to do. It was a safe place from which to hear things and too far away to get involved. He would often run back like a little mouse to his hole and tell Oscar what was going on, but not today. Oscar was madly in love with Millie and thought she shared his feelings. It would devastate him to hear otherwise, especially since he hadn't been feeling up to par lately anyway.

The gossips forgot about Maria and Pastor Paul temporarily in their astonishment over Millie's revelations about men, and while she was sunning and singing and hoping for a man, the old gals inside were trying to figure it all out. Emily had excused herself immediately. "I have an Avon order to get ready," she informed them in her polite, but businesslike manner. But the rest of the group huddled and were befuddled. Millie was an enigma, a puzzle waiting to be solved.

When Bertha arrived on scene, and they told her of the mornings goings-on, she pooh-poohed their interest in Millie. "Oh, she's just an old bag who wants attention. Don't give her any and maybe she'll go away. Where is she now? Not out showing off her wrinkled up old skin again, I hope. If we *could* get that Jacuzzi she wants, at least then she would be submerged!" She was deadly serious, but the women all thought for once she had made a joke, and they tittered as they dispersed. "Remember when she had that sick spell last year and we thought we'd lost her? But, oh no, back she came," Bertha threw that disdainful parting shot as the gossips wandered off to the various hallways. Most didn't hear her, as they were muttering to each other or themselves. Bertha wheeled her way through the Community Room and out the back door.

"There you are, you shriveled up old prune," Bertha said, as she glared at Millie. "You're going to bake and then rot and attract flies."

"Guys? Did you say *guys*?" Millie sat up straight in the chaise lounge and licked her rosebud lips that were as dry as parchment. "Thank you, Bertha, for coming to tell me."

She fluffed her hair and hoped she was presentable. "Are these guys talent scouts or from a studio?"

"From the mortuary," Bertha hissed in disgust. Bertha hadn't changed much after all.

CHAPTER TWENTY-NINE

The Doggie Birthday Party

"The cats will mew, and the dogs
will bark."
—Shakespeare

Maria was steaming as she shuffled through the lobby to Paul's apartment. Luckily, nobody was in sight, or she would have given each one a piece of her mind, and that was scary at her age, considering how fast it was going away on its own! To think that Sarah had started the rumor that she was going to Italy, and it was being gossiped about all over Pear Blossom. "She's on my last nerve," Maria stewed, as she knocked gently on Paul's door in case he was resting.

"Maybe it's time to make our big secret public," Paul suggested, as he tried to calm her down.

"Yes, but that's not the issue here. Why would Sarah tell something like that? I thought we were good friends." She was still fuming and inconsolable, as she continued to tell him how it happened at the hospital.

"Sounds like she made a bad assumption and then got excited about the news and just couldn't help herself and had to tell someone. You know how it is around here, Maria. You tell one person, and you might as well have announced it over Fox News."

"Yeah, but at least there it is *fair and balanced*." Maria believed that quip with all her heart.

Paul went on trying to console her. "You know, Maria, you are going to have to forgive Sarah. I'm sure she just made a mistake and didn't mean to be malicious."

"What? Forgive her? Not unless she apologizes first." Maria was hurt and licking her wounds. "I'm not ready to do that! I may never be ready!"

Later that day, though, after she and Paul had talked it out some more and he had prayed about it, Maria could see that he was right, and that evening when she spotted Sarah in the library, she went in and sat down, and they talked it over. Sarah apologized immediately as soon as she realized her mistake. "Oh, I really made a faux pas. I just assumed, since we had talked about Cat's trip and your desire to go, that it was your big news." She put her hand over her mouth as if to shut herself up after the fact, but then went on. "So, if that isn't it, what is the big news? Give me another chance, Maria. You can trust me."

"I don't have any news right now," Maria clammed up like a tick on a dog's back, and then she changed the subject. "Have you heard any more about the dog birthday party? I've been out of the loop trying to nurse Paul back to health and all. Is it on for this month?"

Sarah nodded her head in disgust. "Oh, didn't you get your invitation? Betty and Gayle have been planning it for a month, and Gayle made announcements with pictures of her dog. They are really quite elaborate. It's scheduled for next Saturday. It's the craziest thing I've ever heard of, but Betty and Gayle think it will be fun. Well, sure. They have dogs, but what about the rest of us? I thought dog parties were just for rich people, but we're all invited. There's a big invitation splashed all over the bulletin board, but I'm so allergic to pet dander that I just don't know if I should go or not. Oh, there's Betty now. Oh, Betty, come here and tell us more about the dog party." She motioned her in and pointed to a chair, but nervous Betty preferred to stand.

She was eager to talk about the party, though. "Well, you know ever since I adopted my little dog Pom Pom from the pound, I've been thinking I should do something really special for her. She is so sweet and shy and probably never had much of a social life, so I've been racking my brain, trying to come up with something that she might like, and then I talked it over with Gayle, and since her dachshund Phoebe is going to be fifteen soon, we decided to honor her, too. You know, before it is too late. Phoebe will be 105 in dog years, and that's pretty old for a dog!" Betty's white curly hair was shaking like a dust mop with all her excitement.

Maria couldn't shut up. "Oh, we can call Willard Scott and get Gayle's dog on *The Today Show*. You know, he honors old people." Sarah was laughing and agreeing.

Betty thought they were making fun of her, but she went on anyway. "Just come and see for yourself, girls. It's going to be a real party out by the garden boxes. I have to go now and talk to Gayle about the refreshments. Ta Ta!"

"Oh, just serve dog biscuits," Maria shouted at Betty, "or hot dogs," added Sarah, but Betty had already boarded the elevator. Maria shook her head sadly. "I think she's losing it, too. I thought Betty had good common sense, and Gayle, too, but now I think they've fallen into the can with the rest of the mixed nuts around here!"

Actually, the dog birthday party turned out quite well. Gayle's daughter brought Phoebe's daughter and her five puppies. The puppies were caged, and they were so cute, especially when they posed for the "three generation" pictures with Grandma Phoebe and her doggie daughter, Lexie.

There was a big, long refreshment table with napkins, plates, and cups with wiener dogs on them. Gayle wouldn't tell where she found the decorations. She said she "sent away" for them over the Internet. She and Betty had been as busy as bees all morning fixing fruit plates, and Emily made some buns for the hot dogs. She only got involved because she loved dogs, she said.

It turned out to be a real party. Others brought their dogs, and Essie even borrowed one for the occasion. A lot of people showed up, some just to see what a doggie party was all about.

As it was winding up, Millie said her cat was having a birthday coming up, so she'd have a cat party in July.

"That would be appropriate," Antonio snickered, as he and Tony were moving the big tables back into the Community Room.

"I have a cute cat story I can tell at the party," but since she couldn't wait, Millie told it to Maria and Sarah, as they walked around the garden boxes to admire the flowers.

"Did you ever hear of the actress named Bonnie La Turner? No, probably not. Well, anyway, she had a time-share with her cat. She would always make her bed first thing in the morning, and then when she left for the day, her cat would sleep in her bed—not on it, but in it. She could never figure out how he got up under the covers and slept with his head on her pillow, but finally one morning she watched him. He just snuck in on the side and slithered up there and put his head right where she slept. When she'd get home, he'd crawl out and run outside. So, she said she *time-shared* with her cat. Isn't that a cute story, girls? Oh, I can't wait for the cat party!"

"Might be fun . . . , but I am really allergic to cats, so you may not see me there," Sarah said.

"How about you?" Millie asked Maria.

"Possibly, unless I've gone to Italy! Ha, ha," she yelled at Millie. "Might as well joke about it, and confuse everybody again," she whispered to Sarah. Little did anyone know that she and Paul that very morning had decided to do the unheard of, young adult, crazy-in-love plan of elopement. As soon as his doctor gave him a clean bill of health, they would sneak away. They'd have to tell the administrator and Maria's family, but just let the Pear Blossom residents wonder and assume and stew and fret—it would give them something to do. Maria didn't even care; maybe she and Paul were becoming mixed nuts, too!

CHAPTER THIRTY

The Bird Woman

"She flies with her own wings."
—Oregon State Motto

Blanche the Bird Woman. Ah, yes, another enigma. Quiet and shy and rather skittish, always looking over her shoulder for something or someone who was never there. No one knew her background of elder abuse, and she wasn't one to share her daily routine, let alone the past. She scurried around doing her duties—washing her small loads of laundry once a week, checking the mail daily, and always looking over the items on the "free" table in the Community Room.

She tried to go out and about when she thought that no one else would see her. She was still collecting coffee cans, but now on the sly. Anyone who would see her apartment could tell that it was becoming an obsession, but she never allowed anybody in—not even her only friend, Essie. They talked in the library at night before Essie watched her in wonder from her bedroom window.

When Sherrie announced that it was time for the quarterly inspection, the Bird Woman panicked. The cans were everywhere! She had tried to stack them and organize them, but she wasn't sure just how the arrangement should be. Alphabetical order—Folgers, Maxwell House, MJB, etc.? Once in the middle of the night, she had discovered that she had the MJB before the Maxwell House in a particular stack, so she had to dismantle the whole pile and redo it. That night she decided it might be more attractive to stack them by colors—red in one column, green in another, etc. When the fears of clutter and eviction took over, she hid them under the bed, up high in bags in her closet, and way back in the kitchen cupboards. It amazed her how many she could fit into an old hat box. The bathtub was full of coffee cans, which meant she hadn't showered in over two months. Spit baths took less effort anyway, but Sherrie was coming the next day for the inspection, so what was she going to do? In desperation, she bagged up the ones in the bathtub into two, big, black garbage bags, and in the middle of the night, she hauled them out the back door to the dumpster and recycling bin area. She had heard the Middleford Waste Management truck there that morning for collection, so she hoped they would be safe there until the inspection was over, and she could haul them back in late at night.

By the time Sherrie arrived the next morning, the Bird Woman's little nest was as clean and uncluttered as a hospital room. There was one package of coffee on the counter, and Blanche welcomed Sherrie in with the invitation to "sit a spell and have a cup of freshly brewed Starbucks with me. It was a gift from Essie." She was trying to be hospitable, but really she wanted Sherrie in and out quickly. The thought of the cans all out of order and mingling with one another gave her the jitters more than the bold Starbucks she was sipping. And then there were those poor lost ones outside, smothering in the garbage bags, and they'd have to be there all day in the hot sun and half the night!

Sherrie dashed through the rooms with her inspection pad and her pen, and the Bird Woman could see her scratching something down, but Sherrie assured her that she had passed and had even gotten exceptional marks for cleanliness. "Although I didn't write it down, the smell of Clorox and coffee actually go good together," Sherrie consoled the worried-looking Bird Woman. "But I *will* have to send someone in to repair that broken blind in your bedroom. That's the only problem I can see," she went on. "You can fill out a "work order" for Tony. The orders are in the laundry room for your convenience."

"Oh, I can probably fix it," the Bird Woman replied nervously, as her hands flew to her chest to calm her pounding heart. "I don't think it is broken. Maybe just bent. I'll fix it," she reiterated. My convenience! Oh dear, what would she do if Tony just popped in to fix it unannounced? She definitely couldn't get her cans rearranged until the blind was fixed.

"Well, okay, but I'll have to check back with you on it," Sherrie responded as she headed for the door. "I hope all the apartments are as clean and as well organized as yours, Blanche. Keep up the good work! Let's see, Bertha is next. Josie Winters has been helping her clean and sort, so it should be easier to inspect this time around. I just hate clutter, don't you?"

The Bird Woman adamantly agreed, as she ushered Sherrie into the hallway. "I'll fix that blind," she told Sherrie for the third time, and she worked on it feverishly the rest of the morning. The cord had somehow become knotted up, which caused the blind to hang at an angle. Finally, in desperation, she cut the knot off, which shortened the cord considerably, but at least it went up and down and was straight. She tried it several times to make sure and then ran up and down the hallways looking for Sherrie. No use to bother Tony now with a work order. If Sherrie could just come and look at it, it would be over and done with. But she couldn't find her, and no one had seen her since she had finished up with Bertha and then Essie's disastrous apartment.

"Well, it's noon now," Bertha told her. "She's probably gone to lunch. You'd think with all the work there is to do around here, she'd just bring a sack lunch, but you know how these young people are; they go to the deli and to Starbucks and talk on their cell phones. How ridiculous!"

The Bird Woman hadn't expected a monologue on the activities of young administrators; all she wanted to know was where she could find Sherrie. Finally, she shoved a note under Sherrie's door. "Come quick! I fixed the blind," she wrote, and around 1:15 Sherrie did appear to check it out.

"See? I told you I could fix it," the Bird Woman beamed with pride.

"Yes, you certainly did," acknowledged Sherrie. "Maybe you could help Tony with maintenance," she teased. "Sometimes he is so over-worked."

The Bird Woman tittered in nervous laughter, but all she wanted was for Sherrie to hurry and leave. She had so much to do to reorganize her apartment and get her columns, her stacks of cans back in some kind of order. Of course, the really important ones were those in her freezer with the coins. Sherrie hadn't seen those, or if she did when she checked for frost and odors, she didn't mention them. Essie had told her it was wise to freeze coffee to preserve it and also that some residents kept their wallets and money in the freezer, so the Bird Woman grabbed hold of that idea. It was good to have some cold cash and coins, even if she had no intention of spending them.

By the time the sun had set, the Bird Woman was exhausted. She had spent the day with her cans. Not counting the thirty-three "orphans" out in back in the black bags, she had tallied up a total of 189 cans. Not a bad collection, considering she'd had to scrounge garbage cans, put up notices, and be ever on the alert for castaways. She knew men liked to store nails in the cans in their garages, and it was all she could do on her nightly junkets not to enter unlocked buildings in search of cans. Her past fears of her sons' abuse haunted her as she darted down dark alleys, and she couldn't venture too far away from Pear Blossom in case she got lost or caught in the act.

It wasn't stealing, just scavenging, she assured herself, and no one, as far as she knew, saw her coming or going. Sometimes she'd walk all the way around the facility, and stand out by the garden boxes, and look at the creek. She began to think about it as *her* back yard.

CHAPTER THIRTY-ONE

Wedding Plans

"Love, to some extent, protects you from age."
—Anais Nin

The Fourth of July celebration at Pear Blossom was a fiasco. For some strange reason, Betty appointed Winnie to be in charge of it, and Winnie had never had any leadership qualities or used diplomacy in any of her dealings with people, so it was a mess.

Winnie said they should have it with the facility on the other side of the creek just like they'd always done. In other words, she basically wanted to pawn off the preparations on somebody else. Betty, on the other hand, thought Pear Blossom should have their very own barbeque. Winnie's main objection was that, "We've never done it that way! We always go over there."

So, Betty put up a survey sheet on the bulletin board to see what the majority of the residents wanted to do. Some didn't care, some would be gone, and some erroneously signed up for both places. Someone scribbled on the bottom of the page, "Whatever we do, let's have a safe and sane Fourth!" Even the survey sheet turned out to be a fiasco, and then it disappeared. When Betty went out to grab it off the bulletin board to tally up the votes, it was gone.

When the Fourth arrived, the invitation still held, so a few strays went over to "the home" across the creek. A few stayed behind, and Betty barbequed burgers and coerced Gayle into bringing her famous baked beans. Millie thought she was asked to bring *condoms,* but Betty said, "No, I said *condiments.*" Millie finally got it right and even brought a bag of cheese curls.

Sarah eavesdropped on a conversation that upset her greatly. She heard Paul telling Maria about Essie's brother, Donald. He had come recently to take Essie out to lunch, and she didn't recognize him. After he explained that he was her brother Donald, she asked him where he had been, and he replied, "Alabama."

So they went out to get into the car to go to lunch, and she looked at Donald and asked him again, "Who are you?"

He told her again and repeated that he'd been in Alabama.

Her surprised response was, "Oh, I just met the nicest man inside, and he was from Alabama, too!"

Neither Maria nor Paul thought it was funny because it showed the decline of Essie's mental health. Paul said he had known Donald for years, and when he confided in Paul, he knew that it was not a story Donald would fabricate. Sarah agreed that Essie was *slipping*.

Fireworks were banned in Middleford, so except for a few bangs and pops of *illegals,* as Bertha called them, it was a quiet holiday. Safe, but not necessarily sane.

Meanwhile, wedding plans were heating up for Maria and Paul. When Cat got wind of the elopement, she became unglued, and her sisters and brother were none too happy either. Oh, they all liked Pastor Paul. That was not the issue. In fact, they liked him so much that they thought that was all the more reason that they should throw a nice wedding for them, and not just have them run off like a pregnant teenager who'd gotten into trouble and had to get married.

"What a thing to say, Cat, and to your very own mother!" Maria was mortified at Cat's outburst over the phone. "Well, of course, I'm not pregnant! Thank goodness I don't have to worry about that! In the first place, I'm too old, and in the second place, Paul just had surgery, so he hasn't been too rambunctious. In fact, I doubt if he ever will . . ."

"Whoa. Stop! Too much information, Mom. All I wanted to say is that we all want you to have a real wedding, and we all want to be there and give you away to Paul." Cat could usually convince her mother to at least toss things over in her mind and reconsider issues, but they had never had a subject like this come up. When Cat got married, she did elope, and didn't tell anyone until after the fact.

"But we already planned it all out, Cat. What if I do change my mind and decide to have it here, and Paul doesn't want to. Then we start off on the wrong foot."

"Well, you have to have your first fight sometime." Cat was joking, and Maria knew it by the tone of her voice. "No, just kidding, Mom, but just go and talk to him, and tell him we want to see you get married. None of us were there the first time when you married Daddy, you know."

"Well, of course not! Cat, what have you had to drink today? Too much Fourth of July celebrating?"

"Nothing stronger than root beer," Cat assured her mother. "I'm just in the holiday spirit, and the wedding spirit, and oh, I almost forgot—my editor set the date for the trip to Italy. I am so excited!"

"Oh, yes, the trip that practically the whole city of Middleford thought I was going on. When is it, dear?"

"We leave the second week in September. Oh my gosh! It's a long way off," Cat bemoaned to her mother. "I can't wait, but by then, we'll have you married off and you'll be Mrs. Paul Clairmont, Mom."

"Oh dear. I hope Paul doesn't think that is too soon. We were kind of shooting for October."

Cat yawned and said, "Well, it's getting late, so run and talk to him and start shooting for August or early September. I thought we could have it at the Little White Church on the Rogue, because that's what he would probably like the best, or we could have it right there at Pear Blossom in the Community Room or by the creek." She yawned again.

Maria was running all of it through her mind at warp speed and trying to visualize it. "I don't think the old, wooden garden boxes would make much of a lush setting, Cat, and there's no room to get a whole wedding party and guests down by the creek. Remember, there's a fence there. Oh, I am so worried. Paul may not like any of these ideas. It's too much to think about."

But, as Cat suspected, Paul thought a family wedding was a wonderful idea. He had tears in his eyes as Maria explained Cat's phone call and the plans that apparently her children had been discussing behind her back. They looked at a calendar, flipped the pages over to October, and crossed out the date they had originally selected. That seemed so final until they turned back the months in-between and looked at the weeks in August.

"That's next month," Maria gasped. It had just dawned on her how quickly the summer was racing by and that before she knew it, she would be sharing an apartment with Paul, sharing his name, sharing everything. She had gotten so settled into the single life, doing what she wanted and when she wanted. Was she ready to give up her independence at her advanced age?

Before she had time to give into those thoughts full bore, Paul was pointing to a date. A Saturday, the twenty-third of August. "What do think, dear? I just sort of picked it out of thin air. It's near the end of the month, so maybe it will give Cat plenty of time to get ready for her trip to Italy."

"If I know my Cat, she could get ready the night before, but, yeah, I s'pose that day is fine. I just hope it will fit everybody else's schedules. That's the thing with it being a family wedding. We have to do it when they can come, Paul." She was looking at Labor Day weekend, which would give everyone more time to travel, but Paul reminded her that often that is a bad time to be on the road or in the air with all the others trying to catch the last gasp of summer.

"You have such good common sense, Paul. That is one of the things I like about you. You try to see things from all the angles, and you try to consider everyone else, too. Now, we have to think about moving, too," she went on.

"Moving? Oh yes, moving. But not out of Pear Blossom, I hope. I like it here." Paul knew Maria was prone to get exasperated with the other residents, but maybe he could help her develop more patience. "My house or yours?" he teased. "You have the best view with the creek and the golf course."

"Yes, but I can't see it, and you have the nicest furniture. I could sell mine, and then we wouldn't have to move it, if I moved in here with you. Oh dear, here we are moving furniture, and we haven't even gotten the date nailed down or announced our engagement! Let's slow down, and I'll go and call Cat, so she can run that date by everyone else in the family, and then we can go from there." Maria started to get up out of the love seat.

"Why don't you call her from here?" Paul said, he handed her the phone.

Maria grimaced as if in pain. "I don't know her number; she is programmed into my phone," and she stood to go. "I should know my own daughter's phone number by heart, huh?"

"That's another thing we'll have to change—your phone number. I must start a list," Paul said as he kissed her, and begged her to hurry back.

Later that day, August 23rd was set in stone as the date that Pastor Paul Clairmont would take Maria Manchini as his bride with all of her children in attendance. The announcement, made by Paul himself on the copy machine at the church, was posted on the bulletin board late that night.

"At least the old biddies will get a good night's sleep before they start spreading the word in the morning," Maria joked, as she helped Paul decorate the bulletin board with gold stars and silver bells she had found in a Sunday School room at the church, while Paul was doing his printing.

But, of course, not much went unseen at Pear Blossom. Essie, who had been watching the Bird Woman tiptoe out the back door, hid in the library until Paul and Maria went to their respective apartments, so she was the first to know. At least, she had read the engagement announcement before Bertha, and that gave Essie great satisfaction.

*   *   *

!!!   PEAR   BLOSSOMS   BLOOM   !!!
Hi Folks! We are announcing our engagement!
Pastor Paul Clairmont and Maria Manchini
Wedding Bells will sound in the Community Room
Right here at Pear Blossom at 1:00 p.m. on Saturday, August 23rd
You are all invited!! No gifts please.
Your presence will be the best gift of all.

*   *   *

"Old age: the crown of life, our play's last act."
From Cicero

Maria wasn't sure about the wording of the announcement. It was too *folksy*—not formal enough, she thought. But it was typically Paul, especially with a quotation at the bottom, so she didn't say a word to ruin his excitement. She had to admit, to no one but herself, that she had been dragging her feet, fearing she was not worthy of Paul, and too old to be starting all over again. But now, the announcement finalized it. She'd never be lonely again.

One day he had said to her when she looked glum and worried, "Maria, are you happy?"

"Oh yes," she quickly assured him. She was just scared and nervous.

"If you are happy, then tell your face," he had responded. "It's okay to show it, you know."

*   *   *

Essie got very little sleep that night. Besides being up late and spying on the Bird Woman, she arose early to catch those who walked their dogs or had a morning drag on a cigarette at dawn's early light. She thought it was her civic duty to alert the facility of the big announcement. Plus, she wanted to beat Bertha at knowing it all—just one time before she was evicted or died, which ever came first. Essie's inspection the week before had not gone well at all, so she was in danger of being asked to leave.

The banter at the bulletin board began shortly after Essie's calls to her friends. Picture this: Six women jockeying for position in the hallway, trying to be the first person to read the engagement announcement. Millie had skipped her hot, prune juice cocktail, which would no doubt throw her system off schedule for the whole week, but when she got the call, she didn't care. She wasn't sure what Essie had said on the phone, and she kept yelling, "What did you say? All I can hear is *bulletin board.*" Essie hurriedly had hung up and gone on to her other calls.

Sarah was sorting her pills for the week, but she threw on a housecoat over her nightie. She didn't care if she was breaking the rules and wasn't really dressed properly. She had to go.

Bertha's shoes were untied, but it didn't really matter. There was no danger of tripping, since she couldn't walk anyway. She couldn't get her house dress buttoned correctly in such a short time, so she threw her apron over her head, yanked it down, and covered up the mess.

Winnie was sound asleep when the phone rang, and although she showed up, she looked a sight—uncombed hair, horrible stale breath, and an outfit of stripes and polka dots. Winnie may have been an alcoholic, but she always dressed nicely and looked clean and polished.

Emily declined the invitation to gather for the reading that morning. She had an important meeting with an Avon client later that day, and said, "I am sorry to disappoint you, Essie, but I just don't have the time. I'll have to catch it later."

Essie advised Betty to stop by on the way to the bulletin board to pick up Maria, and when Betty told her that she didn't think it was necessary for Maria to read it since it involved her, Essie was even more confused and miffed at Betty's refusal. "But, she's on your route, Betty."

"I think she'll hear us if she wants to come, Essie. The bulletin board is practically right outside her door." Betty tried to get through to her, but it was becoming more hopeless each day.

Shortly after the convening in the hallway, Maria did hear a commotion. She quietly opened her door, and although she couldn't see their faces, she could see an odd mixture of colors, and she knew them by their voices. She stood in her doorway and listened to their comments.

Some were positive, such as Sarah's, who said with excitement, "I am so happy for them! They are the perfect couple." Maria decided right then and there that she would ask Sarah to cut the cake or pour the coffee at the reception. "She's a good friend," Maria said to herself.

The negatives were from those who typically had something bad to say about everyone.

"Two old people! It will never work. She is too set in her ways, plus she's a Presbyterian, whatever that is, and he's a Baptist." Ah, Winnie. Up to form; dogmatic and pessimistic as usual.

Maria had to control an outburst of surprise at Bertha's retort. It was so unlike her rude comments and domineering attitudes. "Oh, Winnie, let them have some fun in their old age. They are both lonely, so they might as well enjoy each other's company together. I, for one, am all for it!"

The whole group of women gasped collectively at Bertha's position on the subject, and then, one by one, they began to agree with her. Maria could see the nodding of the heads and hear the acceptance of the whole idea as it started to build within each lady.

"My problem with the whole thing," Essie interjected, "is the announcement itself. I just don't know who Cicero is. See, there at the bottom of the page." She pointed with her long, bony forefinger reminiscent of the stick the teachers used to use at the blackboard. "It is so strange—just one name like Madonna or Oprah. I've never heard it. It's a mystery to me. Do you think it could be Paul's brother?"

Just then, while Bertha was informing her that Cicero was a Roman orator and was before her time—in fact, before the time of Christ—Gayle arrived with her dog. They'd been out earlier for the morning routine, but with all the excitement stirring in the air, her nervous and aged little dog couldn't control herself and squatted right in front of Bertha's wheelchair. That ruined Bertha's good mood and broke up the party immediately.

"That dog needs some diapers. I should have gotten her some for her birthday," Betty lamented to Gayle, as the group began to scatter in all directions. Maria quickly stepped inside and shut her door. She couldn't wait to tell Paul that he had an older brother named Cicero!

CHAPTER THIRTY-TWO

The Heart of Bertha

"Not as man sees does God see,
because man sees the appearance,
but the Lord looks into the heart."
—I Samuel 16:7

After Bertha's early morning outing and then the upset of Gayle's dog piddling at her feet, she wasn't in any mood for Josie Winters to come to clean. But, after she had her coffee and a piece of dry toast, she decided to make the best of it and maybe some company would lift her mood. Josie, after all, was a nice girl, and as much as Bertha hated to admit it, she did almost enjoy having her around, as long as she didn't get too nosy or preach too much. She was good at what she did—cleaning—and that was what mattered, and she didn't have to pay her. A senior project was all volunteer, as Bertha understood it, and Josie would do her best to get a good grade.

Josie bounced in right on time and gave Bertha a big hug. "Have you heard the news? Pastor Paul and Maria are getting married! Isn't that exciting!" Josie clapped her hands.

If Bertha had been standing, Josie would have knocked her off her feet with her enthusiasm. She went on to say that Pastor Paul announced it at church. "And then, just before I left to come over here, Maria called and asked if I would play the organ for the ceremony. I said I would, but I've never played the wedding march before in my whole life."

"How old are you, Josie?" Bertha asked with an uncustomary smirk on her face. When Josie answered, "Seventeen," Bertha said, "Oh, you're getting so old; it's about time you learned it." Bertha actually laughed out loud at her own joke.

Josie could see that this was going to be a good cleaning day, and it was. The vacuuming went quickly, now that the boxes were gone, and then they started sorting the bedroom closet. It was a total disaster!

"I don't like people in my bedroom, and I won't make you change the sheets, but that closet just has to be cleaned out and rearranged. Sherrie said it was a hazard because of all the junk, and she didn't even know I have some cleaning rags and solvent in the back in a coffee can behind the papers, and that's a fire hazard, you know. Oh, and the Bird Lady will want the coffee can."

Josie was continually amazed at Bertha's vast wealth of knowledge. "No, I didn't know that would be a fire hazard, and who is the Bird Lady? Do you mean Blanche? Oh, that fits her! You are teaching me so many things, Bertha. How did you get to be so smart? Did you go to college?"

"Are you kidding? There was no money for that. No, I just have been a reader all my life and a good listener. You know, you can learn a lot by not talking all the time and just listening." As Bertha was continuing to talk, Josie was listening and pulling out stacks of old newspapers. "You can have those if you want them, Josie. Why do I need to save the paper of John F. Kennedy's assassination and the one of men landing on the moon? I can remember those things happening and all the other things in that stack of papers. I just have no room for clutter, and that's what they've become."

Josie thought her dad might like them, so she made a big stack by the door to carry home. Next they ran across some old books. Bertha thought the museum might take them, so they went in a separate pile by the door. "No use trying to sell them here at the next yard sale; nobody buys anything of mine." Bertha was still miffed that she hadn't done well with her sale items that spring. Now she had to figure out how to get them to the museum. Maybe Sarah and Jess could take them. She knew Josie was too young to be interested in old relics.

Stuck in amongst the reading material were extra rolls of toilet paper, paper towels, and boxes of Kleenex. Bertha had stocked up on a good sale at the Food Mart. "Put those in the bathroom for me, please," she advised Josie, and while she was out of the room, Bertha gathered up some loose snapshots that were on the floor of the closet. She was too slow in hiding them in her apron pockets, and Josie arrived back on the scene and her curious mind wondered who they were.

"There you go again, girl, being nosy. Okay then. Just look here. These are my family. See this one here. That is my mama and my grandma, and this one here is of me and my sister."

Josie wanted to correct her grammar and say, "Of my sister and me," but she knew better than to correct her elders and especially Bertha, so instead she injected, "Oh, you have a sister? I wish I had a sister. I've always wanted one. Does she live around here close by?"

Bertha's eyes glazed over, and she turned a deathly shade of pale. "Uh . . . uh . . . I don't know where she lives, or if she is even alive. I haven't seen her in sixty years."

Josie was in shock. "Don't you want to see her?"

"Well, of course, I do, but how could I find her? I have no idea even where to start looking. After she went away to live with *him,* we lost contact. Yes, I know. Your next question will be 'Who is *him*?' I hope you can figure it out, so I don't have to tell you."

Josie nodded her head and knew that Bertha meant her dad. She also figured that, considering how old Bertha was, surely her dad must be dead by now.

"Maybe I can help you find her, if you want. I know how to look people up on the Internet. I'll just Google her."

Bertha had never heard that word. "What? Ogle her? Noodle her? What did you say?"

Josie laughed and tried to explain the workings of the ether world, which only Bill Gates and a few others could even begin to understand.

"Oh, yes, I heard that Al Gore invented the Internet *and* Global Warming. Wow! He must be a smart man. People always say we shouldn't discuss politics or religion, but now we've done both, huh Josie?" Bertha marveled at how smart Josie was for her age.

Josie agreed. "Yeah, I've heard that, too, but how can we share the Great Commission and the love of Jesus Christ, if we don't talk to others about Him?"

"Sometimes I think just being a good example is enough, Josie. Live by example, and don't get me started on that bad example I had to follow! I've tried to be a good person and live a good, clean life, but it's been hard, and now look who I live with—all these nutty old people!"

Bertha was still staring at the picture of her sister and of herself. "Mmmm . . . I wonder if you *could* find her. You have my permission to try. Get that scratch pad over there and a pen, and I'll write down her name. Of course, it could be different by now. She could have married or who-knows-what! But, it's worth a try. Are you sure you want to do this, Josie? To get so involved? Do you have time?"

"For you, Bertha, I have time. I'll just look her up, and if I can't find her, then I don't know what else to do, except I do know one person who does genealogy, so that might be something else to try." She wouldn't tell her just yet that it was Pastor Paul. His Christian beliefs might scare her away, and besides, he was busy getting ready to take Maria as his bride.

"Okay, but I don't want people around here to know what's going on; you know how they talk, and out of both sides of their mouths and all at once, and the worst part is, they get everything all mixed up!" Bertha meant each and every word of that, and Josie knew to keep quiet.

The last things from the closet to go were the cleaning rags and the solvent. Neither Josie nor Bertha knew what to do with them, so Josie started out to hunt for Tony. Surely a maintenance man could use them or know how to dispose of them, and he did, but he wanted the coffee can, too.

"No, that is spoken for, young man. I want the Bird . . . I mean Blanche to have it. She was looking for one the other day." So, Tony shoved the dirty old rags in his back pocket and took off with the can of solvent in his grimy hand. "Josie can drop the coffee can off before she leaves," she advised him, as he loped down the hallway toward the lobby.

"Now, come here, dear," Bertha said to Josie, as she was preparing to leave for the day. "You are an amazing child. I haven't called anyone *dear* in so long and maybe never, but you are a dear to want to help me so much around this dirty old apartment. You know, you are like a worm!"

"One minute I'm a dear and the next minute I'm a worm. Which is it, Bertha? A worm isn't much of a compliment."

"Oh, I meant that in a good way; you just know how to wiggle inside my cold, old heart. Now, get out of here, and go find my sister! And hurry back," she added. She clapped her hands like she used to do at the old roosters in the chicken pen when she wanted them to get away.

Josie bent over and kissed Bertha on the cheek and said, "I love you."

Bertha wanted to say it, but she'd forgotten how, or maybe she never really knew how. "Me too, Josie. Me too."

CHAPTER THIRTY-THREE

Wedding Preparations

"A man is as old as he's feeling,
a woman as old as she looks."
—Mortimer Collins

Hoping that the official engagement announcement would stop the rumors that were dashing through the hallways like a mom in tennis shoes, Paul and Maria settled into the arduous tasks of planning their wedding and their future home together. They should have known, however, that the announcement would only stir up the soup kettle, and more questions and gossip would rise to the top. From what Maria heard from Sarah later on in the week, she thought maybe she and Paul should put an addendum on the bulletin board, so he printed it and tacked it up:

Q and A

Question: Where will they live?
Answer: Undecided as yet, but still here at Pear Blossom. His place or mine, but NOT until after the wedding. So, don't get any ideas!
Question: Who will stand up for them?
Answer: Pastor Paul's best friend, Milford. (Pastor Paul does NOT have a brother named Cicero!) Maria's girls will be in her wedding party.
Question: Will Pastor Paul marry himself?
Answer: No, he's marrying Maria. Do you mean, will he perform the ceremony? No, the pastor from the Little White Church on the Rogue will do the honors.

Question: Are they going to Italy on their honeymoon?
Answer: No, Cat is going to Italy on business. We are going to a place
            called, "None of your business!"
Question: Should we give Maria a shower?
Answer: No, I really prefer bubble baths. Thanks, but there is nothing I need.

Essie alerted the girls once again that there was additional wedding
information on the bulletin board. Some thought it was hilarious, others
were just glad to have the burning questions cleared up, and still others were
miffed.

"Sounds like they're making fun of us," Winnie snorted. "Oh well, I don't
care; I won't be here anyway. They'll just have to get married without me."

"Oh, are you moving?" Sarah asked hopefully.

Winnie picked up on her derision. "Don't you wish? No, sorry to
disappoint you. I have to go out of town. I have some investments coming . . .
But, why should I tell you my personal business?" She snorted again and
stomped down the hall to her apartment.

Sarah and Betty thought their answers were great! "They both sound so
young and happy; It's almost like they are kids! I wish Jess and I had their
spunk. We might do the same thing and get married. He says I look young,
in spite of all my ailments. He feels good, but looks old! Can you beat that?
I tell you true, between the two of us, we really make a pair!"

"Shhhh! Don't say it too loudly unless you mean it, or one of these old,
deaf women will have "selective hearing" and be listening for wedding bells for
the two of you!" Betty said, without a jealous bone in her body. "Of course,
if you *do* mean it, I am happy for you!"

"Heavens no! I don't mean it; Jess and I are just friends. Oh, by the way,
getting back to Maria, I guess you and I are to decide who wants to serve
cake and pour coffee. Which do you want to do, Betty?"

"Emily was asked, too, and she chose cutting cake, so how about if I pour
coffee and you do the punch. Does that suit you? Thank goodness we three
can work together so well!"

The normal activities went on as usual at Pear Blossom through the end
of July and into August. The Wednesday night sing-a-long with Josie at the
organ, the Bible studies with Pastor Paul expounding once a week, and the
monthly potluck drew the regulars.

Millie was pushing for a "Cat Party" right away, but Betty thought it was
too soon after the doggie birthday party. "Let's wait until fall when there's
nothing to do," Betty tried to cajole her.

"What did she say? Did she say she had a bad fall?" Millie was right up in Gayle's face so she could hear, but before Gayle could answer, she tuned her out completely and launched into another plea for a Jacuzzi and a lament over the failure of the boutique to get off the ground floor. "Bertha is right," she went on. "Nothing ever gets done around here, at least not to my satisfaction!"

Sarah and Betty really did want to give Maria a shower, so they planned a surprise party one evening two weeks before the wedding. Trying to keep a secret around Pear Blossom and not let Maria hear their tittering or see the obvious preparations on the day of the shower were not as hard as they thought it would be. Maria seemed to be in her own little world with two-a-day phone calls to Cat, making preparations and plans with Paul, and shopping for a dress and accessories with Jillian. She didn't have the time or energy for socializing with the girls just now.

Pastor Paul was in on the shower, and, in fact, it was his duty and his pleasure to think of an excuse to escort her to the Community Room with an ulterior motive. He told her that they really should give the room a thorough looking-over to see just where the pastor would stand, and where the aisle would be for her to walk down, etc. She thought it was too soon for all of that and stubbornly refused to give up her Daniel O'Donnel show when they could view the room any old day, but he finally convinced her that time was getting short. It certainly was! The shower was supposed to start in five minutes!

"Well, I wonder why those doors are closed. Is there a private meeting going on?" Maria asked, as they neared the Community Room from the lobby. "They are never closed. How odd!"

Just then Sherrie appeared from nowhere, grabbed Maria's other arm with one hand, and opened the door with her free hand. She gently nudged both Maria and Pastor Paul through the door and into the room filled with residents—both men and women.

"Surprise! It's a shower after all, and for Pastor Paul, too." Betty was at the microphone so all could hear. "Antonio, show the young couple to their seats up here in front so we can see them, and then I'll read the games we could play."

Maria was flabbergasted and embarrassed, and Paul couldn't believe the shower was for him, too. They slowly made their way to the front, stopping to greet those nearby.

The crowd was groaning and moaning. "Oh, do we really have to play a bunch of stupid games? I just hate them." Some refused to play and wanted dessert and coffee immediately, but Betty picked up the microphone again, and in her reassuring voice smoothed their ruffled feathers.

"No, these are just jokes that I got off the Internet. We aren't really going to play them; just listen. These were written by Anonymous. I don't know who he is, but he sure wrote a lot of good stuff! Now listen," she repeated. "These are, 'Games for When We Get Older'".

Number One: Sag, You're It
Number Two: Hide and go pee
Number Three: 20 questions shouted into your good ear
Number Four: Kick the bucket
Number Five: Musical recliners
Number Six: Simon says something incoherent
Number Seven: Pin the toupee on the bald guy"

Nobody was laughing harder than Pastor Paul, and later he asked Betty for a copy of those games, as well as for the next list she read. His collection of anecdotes was getting old and stale, but these would really add flavor when he needed to start a sermon or a Bible study with a joke.

Betty went on to read another list by Anonymous. These were: Hymns for the Over 50 Crowd.

1. "Just a Slower Walk with Thee"
2. "It is Well With My Soul", but my knees hurt
3. "Nobody Knows the Trouble I 'Have Seeing'"
4. "Precious Lord, Take My Hand", and help me up!
5. "Go Tell It on the Mountain", but speak up!
6. "Give me the Old 'Timers' Religion"
7. "Blessed 'Insurance'"
8. "Guide Me, O Thou Great Jehovah", I've Forgotten Where I've Parked the Car!

After the laughter died down, and that took some considerable time, as they seemed to really enjoy discussing the games and songs that were so true of their generational, geriatric problems, Betty introduced Duke, the chairman of the Pear Blossom Association. He was called "the Big Wig" around the facility, but not in a loving way. He had accused Betty of stealing from the Association bank account, which was impossible because only his name and Antonio's were on the account. He thought Bertha was trying to run everything, and he did have that right, but it rubbed him the wrong way, and they'd had several fights.

Lately, she had backed off, surprisingly, and let him have his say about things. She still thought he had no concept of correct parliamentary procedure, but Lord knows, she'd tried to teach him. She gave up. Some people are just unteachable, she had decided.

Anyway, he announced that the Association as a group had gone together to get Pastor Paul and Maria a shower gift. He called Pastor Paul to the podium and handed him an envelope. Pastor Paul opened the envelope and read the certificate inside. "We proudly give to you a year's subscription to Harry and David's Fruit of the Month Club. Enjoy your fruit each month! From the Association at Pear Blossom Plaza."

Everyone clapped, and then someone started shouting, "Speech, speech." Pastor Paul tried to get Maria to join him up front, but she shyly refused.

"I guess I can speak for the both of us," he said, as he rubbed his bald head and then stroked his moustache. "We are so overwhelmed with your generosity. Thank you all. You know, it is amazing to fall in love again at this age, and Maria and I feel so blessed to have found each other." He looked away for a moment and tried to compose himself. He thought of his first wife just briefly and then went on. "The Bible says there is a time for everything, and it is time to move on from our past lives and to enjoy each other's company for as long as God gives us together. I don't want to get too long-winded here, so show up for the wedding and hear the rest of my speech!" He laughed and then went on. "But we do thank you again for your friendship and for this wonderful party. Betty, is it time to say, 'Let 'em eat cake'?"

"It is, and you just said it. So, come everyone and enjoy." She and Gayle had the servings ready on a long table, and the punch bowl was teeming with a sparkling, fruity concoction of strawberries and soda.

Sarah was as bubbly as the punch, as she handed a flimsy, flat package to Maria. "I just had to get you something. Open it!" She clapped her hands like a little kid at a birthday party.

"Now?" Maria asked. "Well, okay, I hope I don't spill my punch on it." She carefully pulled the tape off and picked gingerly at the tissue paper. Soon a short, white nightgown was revealed.

"I just had to get you something for your first night. See, it's satin, but not see-through."

"Thank goodness for that," Maria laughed. "I'm a virgin, you know! Ha!"

There were a few other small gifts from special people, and then the party broke up. When Paul walked Maria home, they discovered another gift in front of her apartment door. It was a coffee can wrapped in aluminum foil.

Planted carefully in rich, dark soil was a dahlia in full bloom. A small note was stuck alongside the stem.

"Who in the world put that there?" Maria asked Paul, as he picked up the can, and they examined it. "It can't be from you this time; you were with me!"

Paul set the can on the kitchen counter and read the card to Maria. "A little flower for your new home. Flowers brighten up a place. Could you please save the can for me. I need one or two for storage. Best wishes, Blanche."

Essie had seen Blanche digging in someone's garden box the night before, and she watched her dig up the dirt and the bulb, but Essie decided not to turn her in. "Well, it's for a good cause," she decided when she saw the same can in front of Maria's door. "If I had a coffee can, I might have done it myself, if I would have thought of it," she said to herself. Essie had generously chipped in a whole dollar for the gift certificate, so she felt like she had done her part.

Pastor Paul thought it was a nice gesture on Blanche's part, but Maria wasn't so sure.

"You know, Paul, it looks a lot like one of my dahlia's that I have blooming in my very own garden box, and I'm the only one in the whole facility that has dahlia's." The next morning when they checked, Maria's suspicions proved to be true. The dirt had been disturbed, and a plant was missing.

"Well, at least you still have it; she didn't give it to someone else," Paul tried to placate Maria's anger. "Maybe she couldn't afford to contribute to the gift certificate. She looks destitute, if you ask me. Yes, I know, Maria, you didn't ask me, but let's just let it go. Okay?"

CHAPTER THIRTY-FOUR

Here Comes the Bride

"Let me grow lovely—growing old—
So many fine things do:
Laces and ivory and gold,
And silks need not be new."
—Karla Baker

There had never been a wedding on the grounds of Pear Blossom, and since it was a first, and for such a nice couple, many of the residents went out of their way to *gussie up*.

Some got new clothes . . . well, maybe not brand new, but new to them from the Thrift Store. The women got their hair kinked and styled. Some tried home permanents while others splurged at the beauty salons. Millie worked the gals at the local beauty school until they got her color and comb-out to suit her. They also did her pedicure. She just felt naked if she didn't wear a berry color on her toes, or gold was nice, too. She finally had them do a crescent moon in gold with plum around it.

Sarah felt terrible. The only time that her pedicurist could schedule her was during church Sunday morning. "Don't tell Pastor Paul, but I got up right during the 'Passing of the Peace' and I left the sanctuary," she confided in Maria.

Maria was puzzled. "What is 'Passing of the Peace?' Is it a treaty? A peace treaty in church?"

Sarah laughed, albeit nervously. "Oh no, some churches call it 'holy bedlam,' and it's when we all get up and greet one another. It's noisy. But, the pastor caught me and asked where I was going, and then I lied. I told him I didn't feel well, but actually I went in for my pedicure. Oh, Maria, I am so ashamed."

"Well, if you were a Catholic, you could go to confession and tell it to a priest, but Pastor Paul would say to just tell God you are sorry and ask Him to forgive you. Of course, if that doesn't take care of your guilt, you could go and tell the pastor what you did. See, I'm learning the ropes!" Maria beamed proudly. She would keep Sarah's confidence and not tell Paul, but she knew he would be proud of the advice she offered her good friend.

Oscar and Otis had their blue sweaters dry-cleaned for the wedding, but that was a waste of precious money. It was too hot to wear sweaters in August, so they had nothing under which to really hide and had to wear their short-sleeved blue shirts and blatantly expose their hairy arms to scrutiny. It was either that or stay home, but Oscar didn't want to miss the wedding. Actually, he wanted to see Millie all dressed up, and he hoped beyond hope that the ceremony itself would awaken her heart and spirit to the idea. Even if she wasn't madly in love with him, maybe she was in love with romance, in love with being in love. So, in spite of the protestations of Otis, they shined their shoes and washed their hair in Sherrie's special shampoo and checked each other for dandruff. The monthly potlucks and now a wedding!

A busy social life was still new to them.

Bertha called Josie on the phone and had her come over to Pear Blossom the morning of the wedding to help her. "My care-giver is off today, wouldn't you know it!" She intoned to Josie on the phone. "Could you *please* come for a few minutes. I'll pay you," she begged.

Josie came, but she wouldn't take Bertha's money. "Nope, no money. We're doing this for Maria and Pastor Paul." Josie felt good about putting it that way to Bertha, and she seemed to accept that logic without argument, and after a full hour and a half of fixing Bertha's short, straight hair with the curling iron, polishing her old, black laced-up shoes, and ironing her best dress and fitting it on her, Josie had just enough time to dash back home and get herself ready to return to play the organ.

Essie and the Bird Woman collaborated on outfits. Neither one owned a dress, but Essie had a skirt that she'd worn once as part of a Halloween costume, and the Bird Woman had a top that matched it more-or less . . . mostly less, so they had argued over it for days. The Bird woman finally let Essie wear it because she found a dress on the "free table" in the Community Room. It was way too large, but she duct-taped it and stapled up the hem until it hung from her spindly shoulders like a kite caught on a wire. She forgot to tie the belt, so it looked like the tail on a kite. Essie said they should both wear thongs on their feet, and the Bird Woman agreed, but later they found out to their horror that thongs now meant something else exclusively, and what they had on their feet were flip-flops.

While the residents were preparing and Maria's girls were decorating the Community Room for the wedding and setting up card tables out on the back patio for the reception, Maria was going through the throes of the "bride's cold feet syndrome". "I'm just a basket case," Maria cried on Cat's shoulder. Cat tried to stay by her side to bolster her up and allay her fears, but she was also the self-appointed wedding planner, so she was dashing all over the building. Betty and Gayle were invaluable helpers with finding punch bowls and decorating inside and out.

Meanwhile, Paul was sequestered in his apartment with his best man, Milford, who adjusted Paul's tie innumerable times and tried to calm his nerves. Michael checked on them a few minutes before the ceremony. "It's almost time," he told the men. "Come on down in about five minutes, so you can get up front before Mom arrives. The pastor is waiting for you," Michael said to his future step-father. Michael was giving his mother away to this man, and that was okay with him. He and Pastor Paul had bonded over the golf course in the last couple weeks. Pastor Paul could only ride along in the golf cart and watch. His surgeon thought it was too soon to swing the clubs, but that was fine with Pastor Paul. He hated to admit he had never hit a golf ball in his life.

And then it was time. Josie was playing some appropriate music that Pastor Paul had suggested to her. Thank goodness he knew from experience what pieces she should choose, because she had no idea!

The Community Room was full by 12:50. In fact, Sherrie was worried that they had exceeded their limit, and she hoped the inspectors from the fire department or elsewhere wouldn't show up and tell them that there were too many bodies in the room. All the exits were accessible, and the air conditioner was running at full capacity, so it was safe and comfortable.

At 1:00 p.m. sharp, Michael signaled that the ladies were ready, and Josie began to play the piece they had decided on for the wedding party to enter, and as the strains from the organ filled the room, all four of Maria's daughters, attired in light blue sun dresses, preceded her down the aisle. Josie let her brother, Jake, sit on the bench with her while she played, and he was thrilled!

After a brief pause, Josie loudly played the first note of The Wedding March, and Maria entered the room on Michael's arm. Working through arthritis and other crippling maladies, the residents struggled from their chairs without moaning and groaning. They tried to act dignified, although Millie's voice boomed out, "Thank goodness Josie plays loud. I knew just when to get up!" The Bird Woman nodded in agreement. Her duct tape had loosened, and her dress was sagging over one breast, but she didn't care. She thought she looked the best she'd looked in years!

"Who gives this woman to be married to this man?" The pastor looked right at Michael.

"Her daughters and I," Michael answered without hesitation, and with that he turned his mother over to Pastor Paul Clairmont. Her dress was the same color as her daughters', but a lot less revealing. The scooped neckline didn't really scoop very low, and the three-quarter length sleeves covered up her sagging arms—her *wings*, as she called the skin hanging down.

The ceremony flew by all too rapidly for most, but all too slowly for Maria. She felt dizzy and incoherent, but it was just nerves and not a serious physical ailment. There were no solos, and no ring bearer or flower girl—just a simple exchanging of the vows, some Scripture, and some advice. "Just a simple service," Maria had insisted.

Pastor Paul had memorized his own vows, and he was eager to take Maria's hands in his and look into her eyes and tell her and the room full of friends and family what was in his heart.

"Maria, you know me well enough by now to know that I love poetry and one of my favorite authors of poetry of love is James Metcalfe. He says in this poem what I have in my heart much better than I could say it myself. This is called 'With Heart Sincere'.

> 'I love you, dear, with heart sincere
> And all the soul in me
> I love you more than anything
> That I could ever be.
> I love you for your gentleness
> And for your wistful eyes,
> The sweetness of your phrases and
> The softness of your sighs.
> You are tomorrow's melody,
> The music of today
> And every song of memory
> That time has drawn away.
> I cherish you beyond this world
> Of struggle and of strife,

And more than any other one
Who wants to share my life.
Because you are the faith and hope
Of everything I do,
And no one else could ever be
As wonderful as you.'"

"Oh, my dear Maria," he added and looked lovingly into her misty eyes.

Maria was wiping the tears from her cheeks and didn't know if she could speak.

"Now, it is your turn, Maria," the pastor gently said.

"I don't have any poetry, Paul, but just my own words. You are my friend, and now you are my partner. I trust you to take care of me, to help take away my troubles and my tears. You never criticize me. Your smile and your sense of humor inspire me and bring me happiness. Now I think I can make it through my old age because you will be by my side. I thank you from the bottom of my heart for loving me and making my life worthwhile again, and . . . Um . . . I love you!"

Now it was Paul's turn to tear up. Maria wiped his cheeks with her hanky, and she could easily have gone up and down the rows of the audience and done the same thing. There was hardly a dry eye in the house. Even Bertha had to bow her head and blink back the droplets that were blinding her eyes momentarily.

After they exchanged simple gold wedding bands, the pastor blessed their vows with another poem by James Metcalfe that Paul had selected.

"God Bless Your Vows"

"God bless you, Bride, and bless you, Groom
On this your wedding day,
And bless you always in your love
And every other way.
In perfect health or sickness,
In wealth or poverty,
As much as you have made your vows
For all eternity.
Now give yourself to her, and you
Give all yourself to him,
And do not fall or ever let

Your lamp of faith grow dim.
Believe in him, believe in her
With all your loving heart
And let no jealousy prevail
To tear your life apart.
And may the blessing that is God's
Bestow its grace on you
To sanctify your vows and keep
Your love forever true."

"I now pronounce you man and wife. Paul, you may kiss your bride."

"My pleasure," Paul whispered, just before their lips met, and the audience began to clap.

"I now present to you, Pastor and Mrs. Paul Clairmont."

"Hit it, Josie," Sherrie gave her the cue, and the newlyweds slowly made their way down the aisle and outside to the patio, as Josie played a recessional piece on the organ.

They both plopped down wearily on Millie's chaise lounge and sat side by side. "Whoever said you had to do the receiving line standing up?" Paul joked, as Maria was still trying to catch her breath, but in a few minutes they found some shade and did stand again to greet all the guests and talk to them one by one. Maria put aside her fear of germs for the sake of the day and shook hands with everyone. Antonio tried to steal a kiss, but Paul caught him. "She's mine, old boy."

Essie quizzed Paul as to the best man's name. "Was that Cicero?" she asked, still determined that he must have a brother by that name. The Bird Woman was confused, too. She had no idea that Maria had so many children. She swore up and down that Cat was Maria's only daughter.

The most amazing response came from Bertha, and Maria and Paul talked about it for days. Nobody had ever seen her stand on her two feet, except her care giver, but she slowly pulled herself up to a standing position and gave Paul and Maria each a hug. "I am happy for you," Bertha said with tears in her eyes. "I guess it's never too late," she added wistfully.

"Yep, never say *never*, Bertha. Thanks for your sweet words." Paul never thought he'd be thanking Bertha for anything, but she seemed to be mellowing at times, and this was primo.

With best wishes accepted, cake cut and served, and clothes changed for a honeymoon departure, the happy, old couple whisked out the door around 4:30, destination unknown, except to Maria's family. Paul carried the picnic basket that Cat had fixed for them, and Maria had an overnight bag, more or less for effect than anything else. Since her daughters were staying in town for a few more days, she easily convinced Paul to take the honeymoon later.

They drove north on I-5 to a favorite picnic spot that Paul had been to many times, and as they ate their supper at a table under the trees near the Rogue River, they went over the events of the day in detail. They both heard or remembered different things at the wedding.

"Was that Millie that kept whispering, 'Let's sing?'" Paul wondered in childlike amusement, and his belly when he laughed was as jiggly as the lemon jello that Winnie brought to the last potluck. "It just didn't set up right," she had moaned to the diners who had to practically suck it up with a straw.

"Probably," Maria thought. "Millie has what she calls a *stage whisper*, but it could be heard clear up in Portland. At least she didn't show up in her bikini, but did you see her flirting with the men at the reception? Oscar must have been so jealous; she didn't give him the time of day!"

Paul hadn't noticed Millie's attractions, but he did see that the Bird Woman was about to lose her dress several times. "I think she had duct tape on it. Could you tell? It worried me!"

Several of Paul's long-time friends had attended, and Maria lamented that no one from the *outside* had been able to come to see her get married. "Of course, I don't know anybody in Middleford, but it sure would have been nice if the old gang from the Roseburg Valley Mall could have come. We used to meet for coffee almost every afternoon after I retired. I called my best friend, Marilyn, but she lost her driver's license, and nobody else was available to drive them all down here. I bet they were surprised at the news, though."

Paul assured her that soon they would go up and see her old gang. "I want to meet them, too," he said as he stifled a yawn. "Well, it's been a busy day. Should we head back before we both fall asleep?"

Maria agreed. She too was exhausted, and it was getting dark. She was thankful that the old people liked to go to bed early, so when they thought that the residents were all tucked away in their little beds, they snuck back in and spent the first night of married life in Paul's apartment. He would soon move into hers, though, because he liked the view of the creek and the golf course.

Of course, the night owls who never missed a trick, had seen the activity. The Bird Woman was groveling through the garbage bin for coffee cans, and Essie was up, spying on her, so the secret was out. It didn't really matter. Paul and Maria would show their faces the next morning anyway, but it gave Essie and the Bird Woman something to ponder until nighttime gave way to sunrise.

At least they couldn't see what went on beyond the closed doors of Paul's apartment, which was absolutely nothing! The gossips would have suffered a terrible disappointment. A hug, a goodnight kiss, some yawning, a few words, and then they fell into Paul's king-sized bed, both totally worn out. Maria was so glad it was a big bed, so she'd have plenty of room to stretch out.

"I love you to the moon and back, Maria," Paul whispered in her ear.

"I'm over the moon in love with you, Paul," Maria whispered back.

CHAPTER THIRTY-FIVE

Bertha's Search for Peace

"Give people a bit of your heart
rather than a piece of your mind"
—Helen Beam in *Guideposts*

Only God can change hearts. Sometimes He hits a person over the head with a baseball bat, figuratively speaking. Other times He gently speaks to one's heart, and often He uses another person to do the talking and the loving. Josie Winters was the catalyst, the ice-breaker, the loving young person God used to bring Bertha to a place where she could at least begin to see that she needed the Lord in her life. Josie didn't need to borrow Jake's baseball bat to get through to Bertha. She just needed patience and encouragement and God's strength and discernment to show God's love to Bertha and to show her how much she needed Him in her life.

Bertha had tried for so long to be strong, when all along she was weak and needy inside and out. Her body had failed her long ago, her father had lost her trust and respect, and her family had seemingly disappeared and deserted her. All she had was her domineering spirit, the need to be right and all-knowing, and to boss others around. It gave her a false sense of security and pride. She had no idea that the One who could save her, the One who could give her real strength, and pride for a job well done was waiting for her to humble herself and come to Him. She'd heard the words in her past, but they weren't for her. Her father's sins had ruined her faith. In fact, she had let his sins ruin her life. Because of his failed relationship with her, she was not at peace with herself, and therefore not at peace with others.

She'd often said to herself and several times lately to Josie, "If only people would just get a clue and straighten up and not make me so mad! People around here are so frustrating!" She judged and analyzed and criticized, and it was always someone else—not her—that had a problem.

But in recent days, some things had changed. No one, including Bertha, knew what was going on. A few days after the wedding, a group of ladies, sans Bertha, was gathered in the library. They were discussing the ceremony and analyzing each portion like they were performing an autopsy. Their observations and thoughts had morphed into more than what really happened. Rumors, as they scampered through the hallways of Pear Blossom, had a way of changing everyone's perspectives. Bertha's recent actions were the biggest enigma of them all.

"Not to change the subject of your trip, Winnie, but . . . I'm going to change it anyway. Did you girls see the way that gentleman played up to Millie? I don't know who he is, but he sure seemed smitten with her," Sarah said, as she had been dying to find out about the relationship, if there was one. "Was he a friend of Pastor Paul's?" she inquired.

"Where have you been, Sarah? He's the new gentleman around here. He's staying in the guest room until Pastor Paul completely gets moved in with Maria, and then he'll have his apartment." Betty was as sure of that story as she was that her name was Betty.

Gayle had a different version. "That's not the way I heard it. Oh, sorry to disagree with you, Betty, but I heard that he's related to Pastor Paul and came from up north just for the wedding. He's going back home in a few days." She was as sure of it as she was that her name was Gayle.

And then Essie asked her famous question that ended the discussion. "Is his name Cicero?"

The Bird Woman piped up and sang out a statement that quickly got their attention. "Something has happened to Bertha!"

Millie touched both ears simultaneously as if to turn up the batteries. "What did she say?" She looked toward Gayle for help. "Did the ambulance come? Did I miss some excitement?"

"No, she stood up!" If the Bird Woman could have flown around the room, she would have encircled it and landed in the center of the table. "Didn't you see her?" she went on. "At the reception in the receiving line, she stood up and hugged the bride and groom. It was so exciting!"

"Oh, Blanche, you've really lost it this time. Bertha would never stand up. She can't, and she would never hug another living soul. I'm surprised she was

even there, since it had to do with love and mushy stuff. She is all business."
Winnie admired Bertha for that.

Bertha had been her advocate many times, and they got along quite well,
although Bertha did not approve of Winnie's addiction to the bottle.

"How do you know so much about it? You weren't even there, so your two
cents worth doesn't even count!" And with the mention of money, the Bird
Woman flew out the door and down the hall to recount her coffee cans. The
latest tally in her accounting book showed a grand total of 299. She only really
needed two cans for her coins, but there was no stopping her obsession.

"You know, Blanche is totally correct. I was standing with Jess just
behind Bertha in the line, and she did stand up just briefly, and she did
put her arms around them. I couldn't hear what she said, but they thanked
her, and she sat down and wheeled away. If you don't believe me, just ask
Jess; he'll verify it. Oscar and Otis were nearby, too, and probably saw her
standing." Sarah knew it had happened, and she agreed that it was amazing,
"but it is true!"

"You know, I think Bertha has changed. She seems nicer and more mellow
lately." Emily had joined the group. She was keeping a watchful eye out for
the UPS man and her Avon delivery.

"I've noticed it, too," Gayle agreed. "She didn't snap at me when I
admonished her for taking a piece of cake home with her after the reception.
She's diabetic, and I always try to look out for her sugar habit, and she's always
before let me know in no uncertain terms that it's none of my business, but
the other day, she thanked me for caring . . . Can you imagine that? . . . And
she said she'd be careful." Gayle was still in shock over Bertha's attitude and
response.

Just then Maria dashed by, carrying a bedside lamp to put on the "free"
table in the Community Room. Gayle ran out and nabbed her and implored
her to stop by on her way back home to clear up their misconceptions and
questions. The UPS man arrived with Emily's Avon, so she had to leave, but she
believed Sarah's story implicitly. Maria didn't need to verify it in her mind.

But Maria did verify it in the minds of others. "Yes, it was so unexpected
to see her stand up. I was so overcome with emotion anyway that at first I
thought I must be hallucinating, and then to top it off, she lovingly hugged
us. Not just one of those pat-on-the back, stiff-arm jobs either. It had warmth
to it. Paul felt it, too."

"Of course, it had warmth to it; it was 85 degrees outside," Essie may
not have always known what day it was any more, but she kept accurate

temperature charts in her journal. "Where is Bertha anyway? I'm surprised she isn't in here giving us "Hail Columbia."

Sarah knew the answer to that one. "It's Josie's day to help her. I talked to her myself, Josie, that is, right before she went into Bertha's apartment today. Josie seemed really excited, but she wouldn't tell me what was going on." Sarah tried to pry it out of her, but to no avail.

Maria was anxious to get back to helping Paul move the last of his clothing into her closet, but she tossed in one final thought. "That Josie Winters is one special girl. I think she has helped Bertha in more ways than we know," and off Maria went to let them ponder on that.

"Now, what does that mean?" Essie led the pack into more confusion. "Oh, I know. I bet she is giving her organ lessons! I thought I heard some music several times when Josie was here."

Life was a mystery in so many ways around the facility. If there was nothing else to occupy one's time, a person could lean over the balcony and observe the activity in the lobby, especially around mail-time. Some made late-in-life career changes, and thought it was their job to listen in on conversations, spread rumors, observe and correct, and ask too many questions. It wasn't just Bertha who wanted to be in charge; many were vying for that position, and when they heard that Bertha was busy with Josie Winters, they were ready to submit their resumes to be the boss.

Little did they know that Bertha's life was changing in dramatic ways, and when Josie told Bertha that her daddy had found Bertha's sister's name on the Internet, all the trivial, busybody goings-on at Pear Blossom began to take a backseat in Bertha's life.

"I hope you don't mind that I asked my dad for help. Don't worry; I didn't tell him about your dad or what he did. I just said you wanted to find your long-lost sister, and I wanted to help you, and I didn't know how. Pastor Paul is so busy now with Maria and moving, and I didn't want to bother him, so I asked my dad." Josie was so nervous that she babbled on and on. She thought she should explain all that to Bertha, so she wouldn't be upset. "He won't tell anybody, I promise," Josie went on. "Isn't it exciting?"

Bertha was so over-whelmed that she was speechless. "It's a good thing I'm sitting down," Bertha finally said. "But it doesn't mean anything. It could be anyone. It's probably someone with the same name. Lots of people were named Ernestine back then. Isn't that an awful name?"

Josie agreed that it was terrible. "Was she named for someone?"

"Oh, yes, she was named for *him*. Ernest T. Monrovia. What a handle!"

"That's the name we found! Ernestine Monrovia. She must never have gotten married." Josie was sure it must be Bertha's sister. There couldn't possibly be two people with those awful names. "It has to be her, don't you think? And to make it even better, guess where she lives?" Josie was about to burst wide open.

"Let's not play guessing games. Just tell me where she is," Bertha was beginning to think that Josie might be on to something after all.

"She lives in Phoenix—Phoenix, Oregon, that is. You know; it's just down the road, not very far."

Bertha knew exactly where it was. "I went there once to Wal Mart in the senior van."

"Maybe she's a Wal Mart greeter! Maybe you met her!" Josie was jumping to conclusions, and Bertha admonished her.

"Now, let's calm down and take this one step at a time, Josie. I have to think about this. What is it you young people say? It 'just blows my mind?'"

"Yes, and it's awesome, too! My dad and I prayed about it right before we got on the computer, and look what happened! God answered our prayer!"

"Hmmph . . . well, maybe." Bertha didn't want to give anybody credit for anything just yet until she knew the truth, and it would take her longer to give God any glory. "I guess the next step is to look her up in the phone book, but I don't know where we put it. I haven't been able to find it since we cleaned."

Josie found the phone book under a chair cushion, but sadly there was no Ernestine Monrovia listed in any of the cities in southern Oregon. Josie kept shaking her head in dismay. "Well, she must still be alive, or why would she be on the Internet? It didn't say it was an obituary. Daddy said it looked like she had written an editorial to a newspaper, but I don't know which one. Maybe we should Google her again!"

The only thing Bertha knew about the Internet was how to spell it. She didn't even know if it was true that Al Gore had invented it, but that's what everyone said.

Josie had a question. "Um, Bertha, how come your name isn't Monrovia, too? You said that was the family name, but you never got married, so that should be your name, too. Bertha Monrovia."

"Oh, you're so smart! You put two and two together. Well, I changed it. I hated everything about my life, including my name. I was given the name of Faith Monrovia, and I changed it. I lost faith, in more ways than one."

Josie was amazed! She'd never heard of such a thing. "So, how did you do it? How did you know what name to choose?"

Bertha thought she was getting a little too personal, but, oh well, what the heck? She seemed to be confiding a lot to this young girl. "I went to a lawyer and legally changed it. One of my teachers in elementary school had the last name of Erickson, and I really liked him. Besides, it is sort of a common name—one I could get lost behind. There are probably lots of Bertha Ericksons in this old world. Nobody found me, and that's the way I wanted it, except I did miss my sister, and I still do. This is the first time I've wished I had a computer. I'd look her up myself and so fast it would make your head swim."

Josie was learning a lot of new expressions from Bertha. "I think my head is swimming with all this excitement," Josie said. "How about if I go home and look Ernestine up again and call you and read what I find? Maybe you will pick up a clue, and we can find her in Phoenix."

Bertha agreed to that, and after Josie left, she decided if all else failed, they could contact the authorities in Phoenix. Surely, someone must know of her, if she was still around.

As Josie was going out the front door, Essie nabbed her. "Is Bertha okay? We haven't seen her out for a couple days."

"Oh, she's working on some projects. She's just fine, but busy." Josie was tight-lipped and hoped that would satisfy Essie and whomever else had questions about Bertha's absence. Essie was taken aback. "Projects? I thought *we* were her projects!

CHAPTER THIRTY-SIX

Shaking up the Can of Nuts

Freeze-dried or fresh roasted; Lightly salted;
Cashews, filberts, walnuts, almonds, and peanuts

The lazy summer days of late August and early September found the Pear Blossom residents marking off their calendars in anticipation of cooler days. Except for Millie and a few others, the heat either zapped their strength if they went outside or else they complained about it being too cold because of the air conditioning inside.

"I might as well live in Siberia," the Bird Woman complained to Essie, as her stick-like legs shivered and banged together like two twigs.

"Me too," chimed in Essie. "Why do they have it so cold in here?" But, when Millie, the California transplant and sun-worshiper, invited them to join her on the patio and perch on the chaise lounge, they were back inside within twenty minutes, saying, "Oh, the heat is just stifling!"

Winnie had her beverages to cool her down or heat her up accordingly, and she was out of sight during the day time hours, for the most part. She stomped down the hall with her cane to check the afternoon mail and then stomped back to her apartment. "I have a doctor's appointment," she said importantly every day around 2:45. They all knew it was Dr. Phil.

Betty and Gayle had their dogs to walk and groom and keep cool. They planned the September potluck, the games on Friday nights, and kept putting Millie's idea of a cat party on the back burner. As co-social directors, they bounced other ideas off each other. Maybe a costume party for Halloween, a new design for the bulletin board, or an aerobics class would cheer up the residents in the coming months.

Sarah and Jess were spending more time together now that Sarah didn't have Maria to call and confide in quite so much, but they would never get married as Maria and Paul had done. They just enjoyed each other's company and their interests, as much as Sarah's health would allow. She was still able to volunteer with The Friends of the Library, and they loved to attend the plays at the Ann Miller Theater.

In fact, George Melrose, the new man who had moved into Pastor Paul's apartment, was in the forth-coming fall production of *The Odd Couple.* He had acted just previously in a theater in Roseburg, and when Millie got wind of his theatrical talents, she never again looked at Oscar, Antonio, or any other man. "It's meant to be," she gushed to Sarah. "Just think . . . an actor living right here within these walls. He can help me convince Sherrie to put on our own production, and maybe we can still have a boutique and a Jacuzzi!" Sarah couldn't figure out how all of that was connected, but with a new man for Millie anything could be possible. "What did you say?" Millie asked, when Sarah told her to go for the gusto. "Did you say *bust?*" she asked, as she looked down at her sagging chest. "Do you think I should get an underwire? I wore so many of those under my gowns. I especially remember that awful tight one when I was in the play . . ."

Emily's last Avon order went out on September 20th. "It's just too hard to get customers any more. Besides, I want to spend more time with my grandchildren," she told Sarah.

Emily still side-stepped the gossip and the problems that continued to go on at Pear Blossom. Her blood pressure was high enough as it was without taking on the woes of the world. "There's nothing I could do to help them anyway, so let's just leave it all to Bertha," she said to Sarah, as she went about her business.

Maria and Paul escaped on their honeymoon to Coeur d' Alene, Idaho near the end of September. Paul arranged for them to stay in a condo near the lake for two weeks, and with a rental car, they visited Sandpoint and Lake Pend Oreille. They drove across the border of Idaho into Washington State and visited Maria's daughter in Spokane one afternoon. She took them to the beautifully refurbished Davenport Hotel for lunch and on a drive around Manito Park and a stroll through the Japanese Gardens. Gabby was single and "wasn't as lucky to meet a nice man like Paul," she told her mother. "You make such a cute couple," she added.

About once a day, Maria would say to Paul, "Well, I wonder what is going on at *the home.* Do you think they are makin' it without us?"

"Oh, I doubt it," Paul joked. "Of course, they do have Bertha in charge, to keep them in line."

However, when they returned to Pear Blossom, they found that Bertha was no longer in charge. The residents of Pear Blossom were on their own. She had too much going on in her life to concern herself "with what was Sherrie's job anyway," she told Josie Winters.

"And it's all because of you, my dear," she added, as she patted Josie's arm.

Josie was into her senior year now of high school, and her senior project had taken on a life of its own. She became way more involved than even she had planned, and she had to select the parts of Bertha's life and story that Bertha wanted let out for public display.

"My story will *not* read like an open book." Bertha slipped back into her old domineering spirit. "I don't know what a *power point presentation* is, but leave me out of it," she demanded of Josie.

"But you have become an example of a life that was so messed up, and now the Lord has changed you! How can I not talk about you?" Josie was near tears, but they were happy ones.

"Why don't you just take me in for *show and tell?*" Bertha joked.

"No, that's grade school stuff. That's what Jake does," Josie said, wiping her eyes.

"Now that we've found your sister, you could go on Oprah! She loves these kinds of reunions!"

"Wouldn't want to do that either. But, wasn't that funny when I was going to meet Ernestine, and Essie asked me where I was going, and I said I was going to see Ernie. They all think I have a man! I heard them whispering about it the other day. And they'll never know the truth unless we tell them because Ernie can't leave the nursing home, so they'll never see her."

"Yeah, that's funny, but it's sad, too. It must be so hard to have to stay in one place 24/7." Josie at her young age couldn't imagine the confinement. "At least you found her before it was too late," Josie added. "God is so good, huh, Bertha?"

"Yeah, better than I remember. Oh, look at the time, girl. I promised Pastor Paul I would come to Bible study today. Do you mind?"

"Mind?" Of course, she didn't mind. Josie had asked Pastor Paul to personally invite her.

"She's changing, isn't she?" Pastor Paul could see a difference. "You must really be doing a good senior project, Josie."

"It's a God thing. He's working in her heart to forgive and forget. I think she is even beginning to like herself. Do you know that she went with Millie to the beauty school last week to get her hair styled? She said she hadn't been to a salon in over forty years! She just whacked it off every now and then herself."

Josie left it at that. Bertha's secrets were her own, and God was in control.

Now, Josie needed to see what she could do for Essie. She'd neglected to even look in on her lately. Little did Josie know that Essie's life was so out of order that Sherrie would soon be notifying a case worker, in accordance with her doctor's orders, to find a new home for Essie. Essie had failed the inspection miserably on all counts, and her health, both mentally and physically, was gradually deteriorating. When Millie had reported that she thought that Essie was *tetched* in the head, Sherrie had taken it with a grain of salt, but one evening when Sherrie was working later than usual, she herself had witnessed Essie lining up five fake fingernails outside of Winnie's door. Another day she had a birdcage with a stuffed parrot inside, and she was singing to it and trying to get it to eat. She had been carrying it through the lobby every evening, Sherrie was told. At night she put a towel over the top, and she set it on the free table. "If you won't talk to me, I don't want to sing to you any more," Sherrie heard her say. That was the nail in her coffin.

CHAPTER THIRTY-SEVEN

A Broken Heart

"When Life knocks at the door,
No one can wait.
When Death makes his arrest,
We have to go."
—John Masefield

Maria was happier than she'd been in years. Her doctor said even her blood pressure was lower, and her arthritis didn't seem so debilitating. Laughter must truly be good medicine, and with Paul and his wonderful sense of humor, there was plenty of merriment every day.

"You are so funny, you make clowns laugh," Cat told him when she stopped in briefly on her return from Italy. He was regaling a library full of women after the Wednesday Bible study, and Cat joined her mother for the weekly lesson and the socializing afterwards and to give Sarah some pictures of Tuscany where she had visited.

"You know, Kitten, you fit right in here." Millie gushed to Cat, as she stroked her arm. "Why don't you move in? We need some new blood around here. You could be *a new lady*, like your mother was at first. Well, of course, we do have George, a new gentleman."

Cat couldn't wait for Maria to fill her in on Millie and George. "But what happened between Millie and Oscar? No more trips to the Dairy Queen?"

"No, and it's really sad. I feel so sorry for Oscar. He was starting to come out of his shell there for awhile, and I think he was really smitten with Millie, even though they were so different."

The ambulance came for Oscar twice in September when he had some "funny little spells," as Otis described them. Millie pooh-poohed them. "Oh, he's just doing it for attention. He's still trying to fall for me, in every sense of the word. Can't he see I've gone on to greener pastures?"

Yes, that is exactly what he saw and what broke his heart, and when Otis found him unresponsive in his bed on that frosty morning in October, the medics and then the coroner were called, and an autopsy was ordered. Something was just not right. The back door off the Community Room was found propped open, and when Essie was interviewed, she told them what she had seen, but, of course, she was just a nutty old lady soon to be moving to a home with advanced care. "I saw someone in a black leather jacket late last night standing by the creek. It was leather all right. I could tell by the smoothness and the way the light of the moon hit it. She had a shovel, too." That was all the information she was giving them; she had her alliances.

The detectives followed the tracks of the tennis shoes to what looked like a small grave site out beyond the garden boxes and over the fence near the creek. The dirt was moist with the dew of the frost, and it was easy digging. They held an amber-colored bottle up to the light of the morning sun. "Abilena Cathartic Water, A Laxative," the label said. Nothing too toxic there; just an old bottle, they determined. Digging deeper, they soon heard their shovels clang against something metal, and they unearthed two large coffee cans. There was no rust involved; in fact, they looked brand new. They had large numbers on them: Number 299 on one and Number 300 on the other. They dug around some more, but could find nothing else, so closed up the shallow hole and carried the heavy, unopened coffee cans into the Community Room.

"Oh, are those for the Bird Woman? She collects them, you know," Winnie, who was nosing around, blurted out.

"What kind of woman did you say?" Detective Graham was quick with the question.

"The Bird Woman," Winnie repeated. "Well, her real name is Blanche, and she lives down there." She pointed down the west hallway on the main floor. "She'll be so happy to have some more cans."

The men waited for Winnie to leave the room before they opened the cans. Inside were Blanche's coins, the cold, hard cash she'd hidden in her freezer. She'd decided just the day before that since Pear Blossom was her home, then the area out by the creek was her back yard, so she'd hide them just like her father had done in *his* backyard. They'd be safe right there for a long, long time, she figured. She'd always felt safe at Pear Blossom.

But, as fate would have it, her timing was terrible, and forgetting to close the back door on the very same night that Oscar died, led the detectives to her doorway, via Winnie's help, with all kinds of questions. They soon determined that no crime was committed. The only crime was the loss of the Bird Woman's mind, as she began to recount the stacks of coffee cans for them. She and Essie would both be going to the same facility across town, and that would make room for two *new ladies*.

An overdose of valium took Oscar's life. The empty bottle was found near his bed and inside was a short note. "Good-bye, Otis. I couldn't keep her attention any longer. Please give my new blue sweater to Pastor Paul; he seems like a nice man."

Pastor Paul offered the following eulogy at the short memorial service in the Community Room:

"Hold fast to dreams
For if dreams die
Life is a broken-winged bird
That cannot fly.
Hold fast to dreams
For when dreams go
Life is a barren field
Frozen with snow."
—Langston Hughes

*   *   *

They come and they go. Oh say, did you meet Connie? She's 94 and grows her own wheat grass and herbs right in her apartment. She's from the South, and she speaks three languages. Well, one is only Pig Latin, but nevertheless, three languages! Yes, she's the *New Lady!*